# VALVULAR HEART DISEASE

**Bruce W Andrus**, MD, FACC

Assistant Professor of Medicine (Cardiology)
Dartmouth Medical School, Hanover, NH, USA

Attending Cardiologist
Dartmouth Hitchcock Medical Center
Lebanon, NH, USA

**John C Baldwin**, MD, FACS

Visiting Professor of Surgery
Harvard Medical School
Boston, MA, USA

President and Chief Executive Officer
CBR Institute for Biomedical Research
Boston, MA, USA

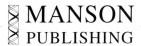

MANSON
PUBLISHING

## Dedication

To Stephanie, Sarah, and Erica, my wonderful family, who give my life much of its meaning and had the strength and generosity to encourage this project.

*Bruce W Andrus*

To Norman Shumway, meteoric genius, supremely skilled surgeon, ironic mentor, provocative teacher, changer of lives.

*John C Baldwin*

**Case studies**
The individual histories described are fictional. They have been weaved together by the author from the recollections of many different patients and some imagination. The intent is to incorporate many of the rather dryly enumerated etiologies, symptoms, findings, and treatment options presented in the preceding sections of the chapters.

**Copyright © 2006 Manson Publishing Ltd**

ISBN: 1–84076–058–3
ISBN 978–1–84076–058–3

A CIP catalogue record for this book is available from the British Library.

For full details of all Manson Publishing Ltd titles please write to:
Manson Publishing Ltd, 73 Corringham Road, London NW11 7DL, UK.
Tel: +44(0)20 8905 5150
Fax: +44(0)20 8201 9233
Website: www.mansonpublishing.com

**Commissioning editor:** Jill Northcott
**Project manager:** Paul Bennett
**Copy-editor:** Ruth Maxwell
**Cover design:** Cathy Martin, Presspack Computing Ltd
**Book design and layout:** Cathy Martin, Presspack Computing Ltd
**Colour reproduction:** Tenon & Polert Colour Scanning Ltd, Hong Kong
**Printed by:** Grafos SA, Barcelona, Spain

# Contents

# Preface

The study of valvular heart disease has progressed rapidly over the past two decades. The understanding of etiology and natural history, the precision of noninvasive assessment, and the surgical and interventional management of valve disease have all improved dramatically. Coupled with an appreciation of physiologic principles, thoughtful interviews and physical exam, current technology allows clinicians to characterize valve lesions fully. In addition, evolving techniques in interventional cardiology and cardiac surgery, guided by quantitative outcome analysis, have reduced the morbidity and mortality of these procedures. Throughout this handbook, we have endeavored to incorporate these developments.

Since the clinician's work generally begins with a patient's complaint, we have devoted most of the first chapter to the evaluation of symptoms commonly voiced by those with valvular heart disease. The second chapter focuses on the evaluation of murmurs, an important topic, since their recognition is critical to diagnosing asymptomatic valvular heart disease before irreversible myocardial damage occurs. The middle chapters provide a structured summary of the current understanding of the etiology, pathophysiology, natural history, clinical presentation, laboratory features, and medical and surgical treatment of valve disease. Single valve lesions are followed by mixed valve disease and an additional chapter on multiple valve disease. The final chapters address special topics in valvular heart disease which are not covered in a valve-by-valve approach. These include infective endocarditis, drug-related valvulopathy, pregnancy, special concerns in the elderly, valve prostheses, and improvement efforts in valvular heart disease.

In the interest of evidence-based medical practice and consistent, rational application of limited resources, we have extensively cited clinical guidelines and recommendations from specialty societies on both sides of the Atlantic.

We expect the succinct and structured text, complemented by current guidelines and abundant images, will be a valuable reference for all involved in the care of patients with valvular heart disease including medical students, house officers/registrars, cardiac nurse specialists, generalist physicians, and cardiologists.

Bruce W. Andrus
John C. Baldwin

# Glossary of Abbreviations

| | | | | |
|---|---|---|---|---|
| ACC | American College of Cardiology | | LVEDV | left ventricular end-diastolic volume |
| ACE | angiotensin-converting enzyme | | LVH | left ventricular hypertrophy |
| AHA | American Heart Association | | LVOT | left ventricular outflow tract |
| AI | aortic insufficiency (synonym for AR) | | MAC | mitral annular calcification |
| ALT | alanine aminotransferase | | MDCT | multidetector computed tomography |
| AMVL | anterior mitral valve leaflet | | MR | mitral regurgitation |
| aPTT | activated partial thromboplastin time | | MRI | magnetic resonance imaging |
| AR | aortic regurgitation | | MS | mitral stenosis |
| ARB | angiotensin receptor blocker | | MSCT | multislice computed tomography |
| AS | aortic stenosis | | MV | mitral valve |
| ASD | atrial septal defect | | MVA | mitral valve area |
| AST | aspartate aminotransferase | | MVP | mitral valve prolapse |
| AV | atrioventricular | | MVR | mitral valve replacement |
| AVA | aortic valve area | | OSA | obstructive sleep apnea |
| AVR | aortic valve replacement | | PA | pulmonary artery |
| BSA | body surface area | | PABV | percutaneous aortic balloon valvotomy |
| CAD | coronary artery disease | | PAF | paroxysmal atrial fibrillation |
| CDC | Center for Disease Control | | PAP | pulmonary artery pressure |
| CE | Carpentier Edwards | | PASP | pulmonary artery systolic pressure |
| CHF | congestive heart failure | | PAWP | pulmonary artery wedge pressure |
| CMR | cardiac magnetic resonance | | PCI | percutaneous coronary intervention |
| CO | cardiac output | | PCWP | pulmonary capillary wedge pressure |
| COPD | chronic obstructive pulmonary disease | | PET | positron emission tomography |
| CRT | cardiac resynchronization therapy | | PHT | pulmonary hypertension |
| CT | computed tomography | | PMBV | percutaneous mitral balloon valvotomy |
| CVP | central venous pressure | | PMI | point of maximal intensity |
| CXR | chest X-ray | | PMVL | posterior mitral valve leaflet |
| DCCV | direct current cardioversion | | PR | pulmonic regurgitation |
| DNA | deoxyribonucleic acid | | PS | pulmonic stenosis |
| EBCT | electron beam computed tomography | | RA | right atrium |
| ECG | electrocardiogram | | RCT | randomized clinical trial |
| EF | ejection fraction | | RF | regurgitant fraction |
| ESC | European Society of Cardiology | | RSV | regurgitant stroke volume |
| ERO | effective regurgitant orifice | | RT3D | real-time three dimensional |
| ESD | end-systolic diameter | | RV | right ventricle |
| ESRD | end-stage renal disease | | RVEDP | right ventricular end-diastolic pressure |
| FC | functional class | | RVG | radionuclide ventriculogram |
| FDA | Food and Drug Administration | | RVH | right ventricular hypertrophy |
| FSV | forward stroke volume | | SEP | systolic ejection period |
| GI | gastrointestinal | | SVC | superior vena cava |
| GU | genitourinary | | SVR | systemic vascular resistance |
| HMG-CoA | hydroxymethylglutaryl coenzyme A | | TEE | transesophageal echocardiography |
| HOCM | hypertrophic obstructive cardiomyopathy | | TIA | transient ischemic attack |
| | | | TR | tricuspid regurgitation |
| IE | infective endocarditis | | TS | tricuspid stenosis |
| INR | international normalized ratio | | TSP | Toronto stentless prosthetic valve |
| IVC | inferior vena cava | | TSV | total stroke volume |
| JVP | jugular venous pulsation | | VHD | valvular heart disease |
| LA | left atrium | | $V_{regurg}$ | regurgitant volume |
| LV | left ventricle | | VSD | ventricular septal defect |
| LVEDP | left ventricular end-diastolic pressure | | WPW | Wolf–Parkinson–White (syndrome) |

# Chapter One

# Approach to the Patient

### General principles

The recognition of valvular heart disease can be challenging. The condition of the patient may range in severity from asymptomatic to severe distress. Moreover, the illness may not be readily attributable to the cardiovascular system. Infective endocarditis may mimic a rheumatologic or neurologic condition, while acute mitral regurgitation may be misinterpreted as a primary pulmonary disorder. Making a prompt and accurate diagnosis, while avoiding excessive laboratory investigation, may test the acumen of seasoned clinicians.

The successful approach to these patients depends upon an open-minded history and careful physical exam, an understanding of the pathophysiology and the cardinal features of each disorder, and the discipline to consider the differential diagnosis of each patient's chief complaint. Intelligent use of a rapidly growing diagnostic menu serves to confirm or exclude competing diagnoses.

### History

As in nearly all of medicine, most clues to a diagnosis come from the history. This should not be compromised. Trying to save minutes at this stage may waste hours in fruitless investigation later.

#### PAST MEDICAL HISTORY

A patient's prior medical history importantly shapes his future risk of valvular heart disease. Examples of relevant past events and the cardiac valve lesions they are associated with include the following: a history of rheumatic fever (mitral stenosis, MS and aortic stenosis, AS); prior episodes of infective endocarditis (recurrent, IE); intravenous drug use (IE); use of anorectic medications (pulmonic stensosis, PS); carcinoid tumors (pulmonic stenosis, PS); long-term indwelling vascular devices, dental, genitourinary, or gastrointestinal procedures (IE);

hypertension or hyperlipidemia (AS); chromosomal abnormalities such as Trisomy 21 (mitral valve prolapse, MVP, mitral regurgitation, MR, aortic regurgitation, AR); collagen vascular disease such as Marfan's syndrome (AS); end-stage renal disease (valvular calcification); syphilis (AR); congenital bicuspid aortic valve (AS); coronary artery disease (MR). Additionally, pulmonary hypertension leads to tricuspid regurgitation (TR) even in anatomically normal tricuspid valves, and radiation therapy may predispose to TR (Waller *et al.*, 1995a). Fabry's disease and Whipple's disease may result in tricuspid stenosis (TS). Methysergide may increase the risk of TS (Waller *et al.*, 1995b). Finally, a history of past valve surgery increases the risk of future valve problems by way of prosthetic valve endocarditis or structural failure.

#### FAMILY HISTORY

Although genetics undoubtedly plays a role in valvular heart disease, it usually does not participate in a simple Mendelian manner. An exception to this is myxomatous valve disease, which may be transmitted as an autosomal dominant trait. For most valve lesions, a positive family history only modestly increases the risk of disease. It is worth recording, nonetheless. In so doing, the clinician may identify a family with a previously unrecognized genetic mutation and allow early diagnosis of relatives.

#### SOCIAL HISTORY

The social history may provide valuable information about predisposing illnesses or habits mentioned above. For example, a childhood spent in a nonindustrialized region of the world greatly increases the risk of rheumatic valve disease. A history of unprotected sex or intravenous drug abuse raises the possibility of syphilitic aortitis or infective endocarditis.

CHIEF COMPLAINT AND PRESENT ILLNESS

The time course for valvular heart disease varies widely, ranging from minutes in the case of a ruptured papillary muscle, to decades in calcified aortic stenosis. Regardless of the tempo, however, there are some symptoms which are repeatedly encountered in patients with valvular heart disease (VHD). These symptoms are discussed in the following section.

*Dyspnea*

This is the most common presenting complaint in valvular heart disease. Unfortunately, it is also very nonspecific, occurring in nearly any disturbance of cardiopulmonary function. Features which are somewhat more specific for left heart failure include orthopnea and paroxysmal nocturnal dypsnea. In valvular heart disease, these symptoms result from increased left atrial pressure > increased pulmonary venous pressure > increased pulmonary capillary pressure > interstitial edema > impaired pulmonary compliance and stimulation of juxtacapillary receptors. In its most extreme form, pulmonary edema, the alveoli are flooded with a plasma transudate (1).

In cases of mild pulmonary venous hypertension, dyspnea may not be the most prominent complaint. Rather, the patient may complain of a persistent cough and be mistakenly diagnosed with reactive airway disease or a persistent viral infection.

In addition, the plasma moistened alveoli represent an environment predisposed to infection. As a result, recurrent and difficult to treat respiratory infections may be the principal manifestation of disease.

*Palpitations*

The sensation of a rapid or unusually vigorous heart beat may signal the development of atrial or ventricular arrhythmias. Atrial fibrillation is a common sequela of both MS and MR. Ventricular arrhythmias are much more ominous and may arise from concentric hypertrophy arising from an excess pressure load (2) or eccentric hypertrophy arising from an excessive volume load.

*Angina*

While more common as the presentation of coronary disease, angina may be the initial manifestation of valvular heart disease. This often occurs in severe AS when the dramatically elevated myocardial oxygen demand of severe concentric left ventricular hypertrophy (LVH) cannot be supplied by even normal coronary arteries.

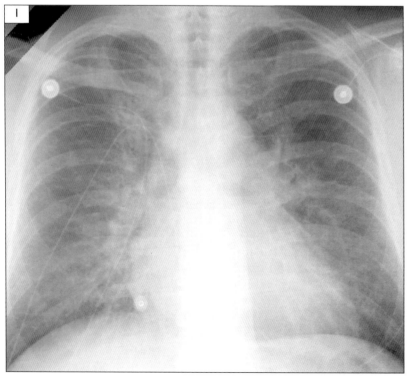

1 Chest X-ray to demonstrate many of the characteristic findings in pulmonary edema, including perihilar haze, vascular blurring, bronchial cuffing, Kerley B lines, and mild cardiomegaly. (Courtesy of Bill Black, MD.)

## Syncope

A sudden loss of consciousness may be the presenting complaint in valvular heart disease. Most commonly, it arises from a sudden decrease in cardiac output resulting from a ventricular arrhythmia. However, in patients with AS, their inability to increase cardiac output in the face of exercise-induced peripheral dilation may lead to syncope as well. Pathophysiologically, this occurs when the 'mismatch' of static cardiac output and falling systemic vascular resistance results in decreasing blood pressure. If mean arterial pressure drops below a critical level of cerebral perfusion pressure, the ascending reticular activation system of the brain will cease to function and syncope will result.

## Weight gain, edema, and abdominal discomfort

These symptoms often occur together as manifestations of right heart failure. As systemic venous pressure rises, plasma extravasates into the dependent soft tissue resulting in rapid weight gain. In ambulatory patients, this is first seen in the ankles and legs. In hospitalized patients, excess extravascular fluid is first detected as pitting edema overlying the sacrum. Concomitantly, the elevated systemic venous pressure extends to the hepatic veins, which swells the liver and stretches the capsule causing right upper quadrant discomfort and anorexia. The lining of the gut often becomes edematous as well, resulting in impaired absorption or oral medications including diuretics.

## Constitutional symptoms

In especially challenging cases, the presenting symptoms may be nonspecific, limited to malaise due to diminished cardiac output, fever, and weight loss.

## Embolic phenomena

A dreaded manifestation of valvular heart disease is stroke or peripheral embolism due to ejection of an atrial clot. This most often occurs in atrial fibrillation associated with MR and MS (3).

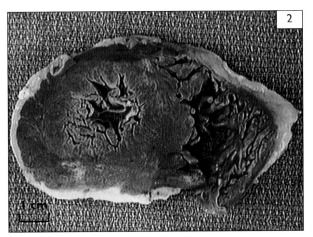

**2** Pathologic specimen of a heart from a female with both severe atherosclerotic coronary artery disease and severe calcific aortic stenosis. (Courtesy of Tom Farrell, MD.)

**3** Pathologic specimen with a right frontal cerebral infarct that occurred in the context of nonbacterial thrombotic endocarditis, and probably represents an embolic phenomenon. (Courtesy of Tom Farrell, MD.)

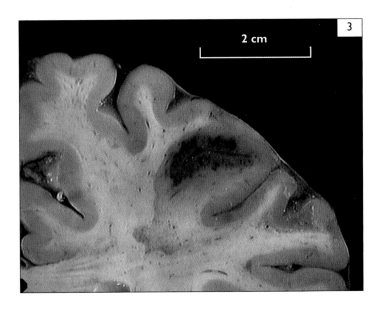

## Physical exam

### GENERAL APPEARANCE

Much valuable information is gathered from the initial appearance of the patient, even from the distance of the patient's doorway. Important signs include the toxic appearance of acute infection, the muscle wasting of cardiac cachexia, the distressed facial expression, wet cough, accessory muscle use, upright posture, and diaphoresis of pulmonary edema, and the cool skin characteristic of hypoperfusion.

### VITAL SIGNS

Tachycardia often represents an attempt to maintain a normal cardiac output or normal blood pressure in the face of a drop in stroke volume or systemic vascular resistance. Alternatively, it may result from hypoxemia or circulating mediators of inflammation. An increased pulse pressure suggests aortic insufficiency, severe hypotension suggests circulatory collapse, and severe hypertension often accompanies acute congestive heart failure.

### SKIN AND MUCOSA

Cyanosis of the lips (central cyanosis) suggests inadequate oxygenation, while cyanosis of the digits (peripheral cyanosis) suggests impaired perfusion. Cold sweat implies hypoperfusion with severe sympathetic activation, while warm diaphoretic skin usually implies systemic infection. Other skin findings may suggest left-sided infective endocarditis. These include tender subcutaneous nodules in the pulp of the digits (Osler nodes), painless red macular lesions of the palms and soles (Janeway lesions), conjunctive petechia, and linear subungal hematomas (splinter hemorrhages) (**4**).

### CENTRAL VENOUS PULSATIONS

Jugular venous pulsation and mean central venous pressure (CVP) are often abnormal in valvular heart disease. In most cases, right heart failure is secondary to left-sided valve disease causing left heart failure. However, in some instances, right heart failure may arise from right-sided valve lesions. In severe TR, giant c-v waves and a pulsatile liver are usually present. Less direct clues to the level of right atrial pressure include the presence of pedal edema in an ambulatory patient, sacral edema or anasarca in a hospitalized patient, tender hepatomegaly, eccymoses (from hepatic synthetic dysfunction), hepatojugular reflux, and ascites.

### ARTERIAL PULSE

The volume, contour, and auscultatory findings of peripheral pulses can also provide important clues to the presence of valvular heart disease. These findings will be discussed in subsequent chapters in association with specific valvular abnormalities.

### PRECORDIAL PALPATION

A right ventricular lift with thrill may betray pulmonic stenosis hidden below. A left ventricle dilated from chronic aortic regurgitation may shift the apical impulse laterally and expand the diameter beyond 3 cm (Eilen *et al.*, 1983). Left ventricular hypertrophy caused by AS may produce an apical impulse sustained throughout systolic ejection. Coupled with a left parasternal retraction, this may yield a rocking motion of the precordium (Braunwald and Perloff, 2001).

### CARDIAC AUSCULTATION

The auscultatory findings will be highlighted as each valvular abnormality is described in subsequent chapters. However, some general comments are appropriate in this section. Throughout the 19th and much of the 20th century, clinicians had to rely on the clinical skills of history taking and physical exam to make diagnoses and form judgements about prognosis. Acumen in these skills separated the master clinicians from the pedestrian practitioners. Perhaps more than any other, there developed a great

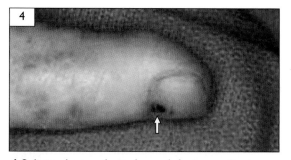

**4** Splinter hemorrhage (arrow) from a patient who died from complications of infective endocarditis. Note the linear subungal discoloration. (Courtesy of Nora Ratcliff, MD.)

library of clinical findings in cardiac auscultation, both extra heart sounds and murmurs. (Hanna and Silverman, 2002). Chapter 2 will focus entirely on cardiac murmurs since they are so often the first indication of significant valvular heart disease. Much attention has been focused on the apparent loss of these skills within the profession in an era of relatively easy, but expensive, access to 'high tech' tools (Schneiderman, 2001). However, auscultation is a technical skill like any other and improves with repetition (Barrett *et al.*, 2004). Therefore, students and physicians-in-training reading this text should not lose heart, but rather, should apply themselves diligently to acquire these valuable bedside skills. Listening to patients before and after echocardiographic findings are known is particularly helpful.

CHEST EXAM

Intercostal retractions, accessory muscle use, inspiratory crackles, wheezing, and evidence of pleural effusions may all be important signs of valvular disease.

## Laboratory investigations

ELECTROCARDIOGRAPHY

As a result of its long history of use, there is an extensive literature of electrocardiographic findings in valvular disease. This experience, together with its low cost and accessibility, make it a valuable tool. Its principal value derives from its demonstration of chamber enlargement, ventricular hypertrophy, and associated arrhythmias (5). The characteristic findings associated with specific valve lesions will be discussed and displayed in subsequent chapters.

CHEST RADIOGRAPHY

Chest films may provide valuable clues regarding valvular heart disease. Pulmonary vascular congestion, chamber enlargement, valvular calcification, and type and position of prosthetic valve may all be ascertained with plain radiographs. Comparing changes over time is particularly helpful; hence obtaining previous studies can be very valuable.

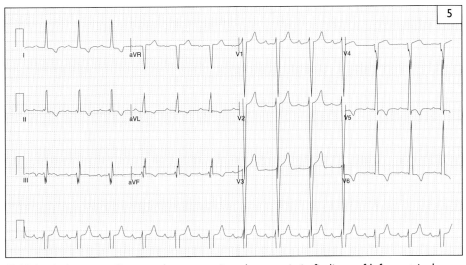

**5** 12-lead electrocardiogram demonstrating characteristic findings of left ventricular hypertrophy which often accompanies aortic stenosis. Note the increased voltage with repolarization changes and widened QRS duration. (Courtesy of Frances DeRook, MD.)

ECHOCARDIOGRAPHY

Echocardiography is the most valuable tool in valvular disease due to its portability, ease of use, safety, modest cost, steadily improving resolution, and ability to assess hemodynamics. Echocardiography began as a simple 'depth finder' which when plotted against time provided what is now known as 'M-mode'. Although this original mode provides tremendous temporal resolution useful for character-izing the rapid movements of intracardiac structures, it did not produce a familar image of the heart. There are now many additional ultrasound-based modalities which provide information about cardiac anatomy, cardiac function, and hemodynamics. These modalities include two dimensional (2D) or B-mode echocardiography in which sound waves are transmitted in a fan-like distribution, yielding a real time, wedge-shaped tomographic image of the heart. Doppler eachocardiography takes advantage of the change in pitch in sound waves which return after striking a moving object. As quantified by the Doppler shift equation, sound waves striking an approaching object will be compressed and become higher in frequency or pitch, while those striking a receding object will become rarified and assume a lower frequency. A commonly cited example of this is the change in pitch of a train whistle as it passes by. In echocardiography, the instrument estimates the velocity of flow in the heart and great vessels by bouncing ultrasound waves off red blood cells and measuring the change in frequency.

There are three subtypes of Doppler ultrasound. In continuous wave Doppler, all velocities along a continuous line through the heart are displayed as a spectrum over time. In pulse wave Doppler, a sample volume is placed on a 2D image and the spectral display of velocities represents the blood flow velocities in this region only. In color flow Doppler, the velocity of red blood cells across a 2D region is determined. The velocity of cells in each pixel of the image are color coded and this information is superimposed on a 2D or B-mode echocardiographic image (6). Tissue Doppler is yet another form of Doppler echocardiography which measures the velocity of anatomic structures rather than red blood cells; it currently has very limited application in valvular heart disease and won't be mentioned in this text. Echocardiographic assessments of valve area, pressure gradients, chamber size, and valve mor-phology will be central to evaluation of many condi-tions discussed in this book.

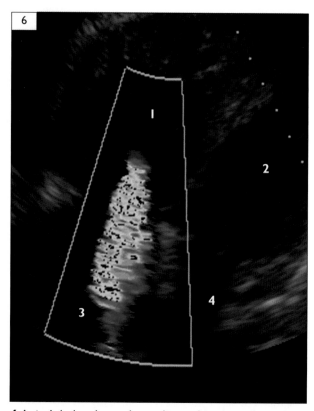

**6** Apical 4-chamber echocardiographic view of a patient with tricuspid valve disease. The color flow Doppler imaging demonstrates the regurgitant flow through the tricuspid valve. 1: right ventricle; 2: left ventricle; 3: right atrium; 4: left atrium.

Because of their ubiquitous use, it is worthwhile to present some details of eachocardiographic hemo-dynamic assessment. Firstly, the pressure gradient across a valve or between two chambers can be estimated by taking advantage of the relationship between pressure (P) and velocity (v) as described in the Bernoulli equation. In cardiology, a modified (simplified) version of this equation is used, namely $P = 4v^2$. As an example, a velocity of 5 msec across the aortic valve translates to a peak instaneous pressure gradient of $(4 \times 5^2)$ or 100 mmHg (13.3 kPa).

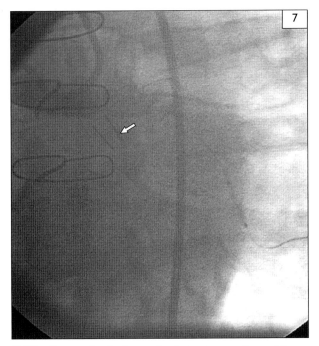

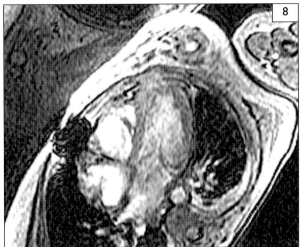

**8** Magnetic resonance image of a mitral valve seen during diastole in long axis. (Courtesy of J. Pearlman, MD, PhD, ME.)

**7** Bileaflet mechanical prosthesis in the aortic position seen in profile during a percutaneous coronary intervention. Note the nearly parallel orientation of the two leaflets (arrow).

Another commonly used physical principle used in echocardiography is the conservation of flow. This states the obvious fact that in a conduit with ends of different diameter, the flow of fluid through one end must match flow through the other end. Since flow equals the product of orifice area and flow velocity, this principle can be stated as $\text{Area}_1 \times \text{Velocity}_1 = \text{Area}_2 \times \text{Velocity}_2$. This is specifically used in the determination of aortic valve area where the first area is the outflow tract, the first velocity is that through the outflow tract, the second velocity is that through the stenotic aortic valve, and the second area is the one unknown which is determined by measuring the other three variables. A variation of this involves substituting velocity time integral (VTI), the distance traveled by a red blood cell during systole, for velocity. This generally yields more reproducible information.

Another hemodynamic measure important in valvular heart diseases is the rate of pressure equilibration between two chambers (e.g. pressure half-time, deceleration time). The chapters on specific valve lesions will make reference to these measurements.

CARDIAC CATHETERIZATION AND CONTRAST RADIOGRAPHY

Although increasingly supplanted by echocardiography, direct measure of intracardiac pressures, ventriculography, aortography, and assessment of coronary vessels prior to valve surgery all continue to play a role in the evaluation of valvular heart disease. In addition, the opening angle of mechanical valve prostheses can be measured precisely in the catheterization laboratory (7). Finally, balloon valvotomy serves an important therapeutic role in mitral, and occasionally, aortic stenosis.

MAGNETIC RESONANCE IMAGING/COMPUTED TOMOGRAPHY

The complex and rapid movement of the heart has limited the application of these imaging techniques until recently. However, recent advances have made magnetic resonance imaging (MRI) and computed tomography (CT) practical, although expensive, means of imaging difficult patients (8).

## NUCLEAR CARDIOLOGY

Single photon emission computer tomography (SPECT) imaging with data pooled from many cardiac cycles (gating) can provide precise measurements of ejection fraction (EF) and chamber dimensions. However, it currently plays only a limited role in valvular heart disease (9).

## POSITRON EMISSION TOMOGRAPHY

Positron emission tomography (PET) is an emerging imaging technique which allows improved resolution and more flexibility than SPECT, including the possibility of imaging metabolic substrates and neural transmitters. In light of its expense and dependency upon mostly cyclotron-produced isotopes, its role in valvular heart disease remains to be determined.

## References

Barrett MJ, Lacey CS, Sekara AE, Linden EA, Gracely EJ (2004). Mastering cardiac murmurs: the power of repetition. *Chest* **126**(2):470–475.

Braunwald E, Perloff JK (2001). Physical examination of the heart and circulation. In: *Heart Disease: A Textbook of Cardiovascular Medicine.* E Braunwald, DP Zipes, P Libby (eds). WB Saunders, Philadelphia.

Eilen SD, Crawford MH, O'Rourke RA (1983). Accuracy of precordial palpitation for detecting increased left ventricular volume. *Annals of Internal Medicine* **99**:628.

Hanna IR, Silverman ME (2002). A history of cardiac auscultation and some of its contributors. *American Journal of Cardiology* **90**(3):259–267.

Schneiderman H (2001). Cardiac auscultation and teaching rounds: how can cardiac auscultation be resuscitated? *American Journal of Medicine* **110**(3):233–235.

Waller BF, Howard J, Fess S (1995a). Pathology of tricuspid valve stenosis and pure tricuspid regurgitation: part III. *Clinical Cardiology* **18**:225–230.

Waller BF, Howard J, Fess S (1995b). Pathology of tricuspid valve stenosis and pure tricuspid regurgitation: part I. *Clinical Cardiology* **18**:97–102.

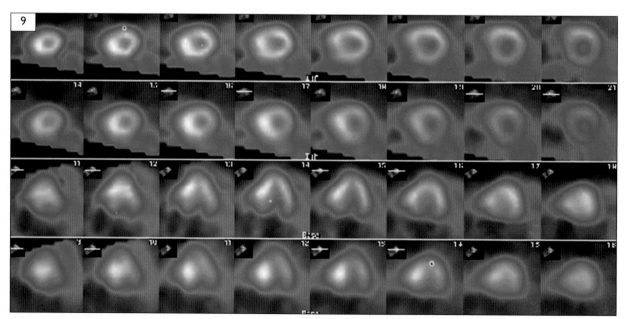

**9** Short axis and horizontal long axis cardiac perfusion scintigraphic images demonstrating dramatic septal hypertrophy in a young female.

# Chapter Two

# Cardiac Murmurs

## Introduction

In most patients, suspicion of valvular heart disease arises from the finding of a murmur. Frequently, this is an incidental finding in a healthy individual or a patient with no symptoms referable to the cardio-vascular system. It is important to reassure patients that a murmur is not synonymous with heart disease. Murmurs represent turbulent blood flow which may result from several possible conditions. These include: (i) increased flow secondary to anemia, fever, pregnancy, or a hyperadrenergic state; (ii) accelerated flow through a restricted orifice; (iii) forward flow through a normal valve into a dilated receiving chamber; (iv) regurgitant flow through a leaking valve; or (v) abnormal shunting between two chambers. In an unselected population, most systolic murmurs are physiologic, caused by conditions of increased blood flow (Shaver, 1995). By evaluating both the characteristics of the murmur and its context, the physician can usually distinguish the potentially serious from the innocent.

## Classification

Traditionally, murmurs have been described along seven parameters in the following order: intensity, pitch, contour, timing, location, radiation, and response to maneuvers (e.g. a II/VI, high pitched, decrescendo, early diasystolic murmur located at the left lower sternal border, radiating to the apex, heard best with the patient leaning forward at end expiration). Physicians with a poetic bent may liken the murmur to a familiar sound (e.g. 'like the sound of air leaking from a torn bellows'). Of these parameters, timing is probably the most useful characteristic. Timing is usually easy to establish by simultaneous palpation of the carotid pulse. In the past, phonocardiograms were widely employed to confirm the timing and contour of murmurs, but have essentially disappeared from clinical practice and hence are no longer available to arbitrate bedside disagreements. However, some stethoscope manufacturers have recently begun marketing stethoscopes with this feature, so a return of this display may be seen in the future (10). In the meantime, echocardiography is widely employed to resolve clinical uncertainty.

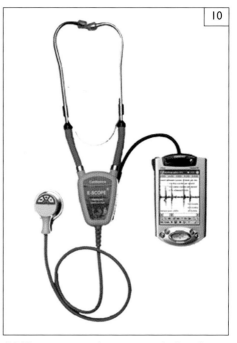

**10** Electronic stethoscope with digital phonographic capability. (Stethographics Inc., Boston, MA, with permission.)

The physiologic basis of murmurs is best understood by reference to the Wigger cycle, a graphic display of simultaneous pressure relationships in the left atrium (LA), left ventricle ( LV), and aorta (**11, 12**). This display will be used repeatedly to illustrate specific valve abnormalities.

A simplified approach to the origin of cardiac murmurs is presented in **13**. A more comprehensive approach is discussed below.

### Systolic murmurs

By definition, these sounds begin on or after $S_1$ and end by $A_2$ or $P_2$, depending on their side of origin ($P_2$ if right-sided; $A_2$ if left-sided). To narrow the broad differential diagnosis of systolic murmurs, it helps to further localize them within systole as outlined in the following sections.

### Early systolic murmurs

These uncommon decrescendo murmurs begin with $S_1$ and end in midsystole. Three lesions create this murmur: (i) acute mitral regurgitation (MR), where regurgitant flow ceases in midsystole because of the rapid pressure rise in a noncompliant left atrium; (ii) tricuspid regurgitation (TR) without pulmonary hypertension, where pressure equalization between the right ventricle and the right atrium occurs by midsystole; (iii) ventricular septal defects (VSDs) of two varieties; a very small restrictive VSD (**14**) and a large VSD accompanied by pulmonary hypertension. The latter two both yield soft, high pitched murmurs (Perloff, 1994).

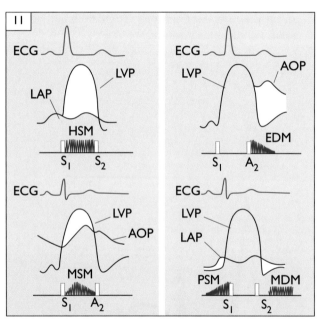

**11** Wigger diagram of invasive hemodynamic tracings with simultaneous display of electrocardiogram and phonocardiogram of common murmurs. AOP: aortic pressure; ECG: electrocardiogram; EDM: end-diastolic murmur; HSM: holosystolic murmur; LAP: left atrial pressure; LVP: left ventricular pressure; MDM: mid-diastolic murmur; MSM: midsystolic murmur; PSM: postsystolic murmur. (Adapted from O'Rourke R, Braunwald E (2001). Physical exam of the cardiovascular system. In: *Harrison's Principles of Internal Medicine*, 15th edn. E Braunwald, AS Fauci, KJ Isselbacher, *et al.* (eds). McGraw-Hill, New York, pp. 1255–1262.)

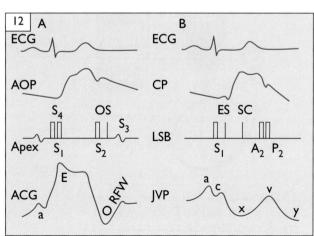

**12** Simultaneous display of electrocardiogram, peripheral pulses, apex cardiogram, and phonocardiogram of common heart sounds. ACG: apex cardiogram; AOP: aortic pressure; Apex: apex phonocardiogram; CP: carotid pulse; ECG: electrocardiogram; ES: ejection sound; JVP: jugular venous pressure; LSB: left sternal border phonocardiogram; O: opening point; OS: opening snap; RFW: rapid filling wave. (Adapted from O'Rourke R, Braunwald E (2001). Physical exam of the cardiovascular system. In: *Harrison's Principles of Internal Medicine*, 15th edn. E Braunwald, AS Fauci, KJ Isselbacher, *et al.* (eds). McGraw-Hill, New York, pp. 1255–1262.)

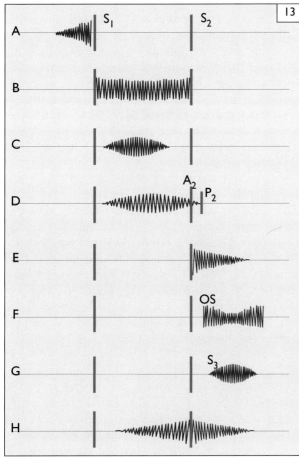

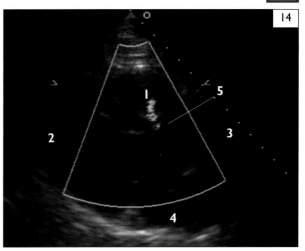

**14** Doppler color imaging in the parasternal long axis demonstrating a ventricular septal defect high in the septum (arrow) with left-to-right flow. 1: right ventricle; 2: left ventricle; 3: ascending aorta; 4: left atrium; 5: membranous VSD.

**13** Diagram depicting principal heart murmurs. **A:** Presystolic murmur of mitral or tricuspid stenosis. **B:** Holosystolic (pansystolic) murmur of mitral or tricuspid regurgitation or of ventricular septal defect. **C:** Aortic ejection murmur beginning with an ejection click and fading before the second heart sound. **D:** Systolic murmur in pulmonic stenosis spilling through the aortic second sound, pulmonic valve closure being delayed. **E:** Aortic or pulmonary regurgitant murmur. **F:** Long diastolic murmur of mitral stenosis following the opening snap. **G:** Short mid-diastolic inflow murmur following a third heart sound. **H:** Continuous murmur of patent ductus arteriosus. (Adapted from O'Gara PT, Braunwald E (2001). Approach to the patient with a heart murmur. In: *Harrison's Principles of Internal Medicine*, 15th edn. E Braunwald, AS Fauci, KJ Isselbacher, *et al.* (eds). McGraw-Hill, New York, pp. 207–211.)

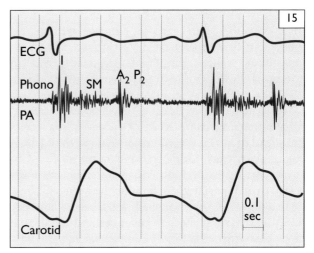

**15** Innocent flow murmur in a young healthy male. Note the short duration and early peak intensity of the systolic murmur. ECG: electrocardiogram; PA: pulmonary area; Phono: phonocardiogram; SM: systolic murmur. (Adapted from Tavel ME (1972) *Clinical Phonocardiography and External Pulse Recording*. Yearbook Medical Publishers, Chicago.)

*Midsystolic murmurs*

By definition, these murmurs begin after $S_1$ and end before $S_2$. Five general conditions produce murmurs with this timing: (i) obstruction of ventricular outflow; (ii) aortic or pulmonary trunk dilatation; (iii) accelerated systolic ejection; (iv) some cases of MR; and (v) innocent murmurs (Braunwald and Perloff, 2001). The frequent diamond-shaped contour of these murmurs reflects the rate of flow during ventricular systole (**15**). These five subtypes will be discussed in turn.

Murmurs caused by obstructed flow may arise from a supravalvular, valvular, or subvalvular location. The valvular causes will be specifically discussed in subsequent chapters. Supravalvular obstruction is caused by pulmonary artery stenosis, supravalvular aortic stenosis, and coarctation of the aorta. Infravalvular causes include infundibular stenosis in tetralogy of Fallot, and hypertrophic obstructive cardiomyopathy (HOCM). Right-sided murmurs are generally recognized by their augmentation with inspiration, while left-sided murmurs become softer with inspiration. Fibrocalcific aortic stenosis may produce two distant murmurs from the same lesion: a coarse, harsh murmur at the right upper sternal border arising from turbulent flow beyond the valve, and a pure musical murmur heard at the apex attributed to high frequency vibrations of the valve cusps. This characteristic murmur bears the name of the French physician who first described it (Gallavardin and Pauper-Ravault, 1925).

Murmurs arising from flow into a dilated conduit occur on the left side in ascending aortic aneurysms associated with syphilis or Marfan's syndrome; on the right side they are heard in patients with dilated pulmonary arteries associated with atrial septal defects and large left-to-right shunts. Murmurs due to increased flow are heard in anemia, fever, thyrotoxicosis, pregnancy, or a hyperadrenergic state.

In ischemic heart disease, left ventricular dilatation or impaired contractility of the papillary muscles may lead to mitral regurgitation. This form of MR is yet another source of midsystolic murmurs.

Several forms of innocent, midsystolic murmurs exist. A Still murmur is commonly heard in children; it is a short, medium pitched, buzzing or vibratory murmur, heard at the left lower sternal border and apex and attributed to vibrations emanating from a left ventricular false tendon or the base of the pulmonary leaflets (Joffe, 1992). In children, young adults, and those with a reduced anterior–posterior chest dimension, vibration of a normal pulmonary trunk causes another innocent murmur. It is less musically pure than a Still murmur (De Leon et al., 1965). Lastly, aortic sclerosis, a senile thickening of the aortic cusps, also produces an innocent murmur (Perloff, 1994). It is important to emphasize all innocent murmurs are midsystolic and less than grade III/VI in intensity. Conversely, all diastolic murmurs and all murmurs exceeding grade II/VI must be considered potentially pathologic and should prompt further inquiry (O'Rourke, 1998; Shry et al., 2001).

Although the traditional hallmark of aortic regurgitation (AR) is a diastolic murmur, diastolic murmurs are more difficult to hear, especially if the examiner does not suspect them. A recent study comparing the auscultatory findings of non-cardiologists to echocardiography revealed that a diastolic murmur was heard in only 14% of patients with moderate AR, but a systolic murmur due to increased total stroke volume was heard in 86% (Heidenreich et al., 2004).

*Late systolic murmurs*
The principal source of murmurs with this timing is mitral valve prolapse with regurgitation. The murmur is typically preceded by one or more midsystolic clicks. At the diminished ventricular volume produced by standing or Valsalva strain, prolapse occurs earlier, lengthening and softening the murmur. With the increased filling of squatting, prolapse occurs later, hence the click moves towards $S_2$ and the murmur is shorter and louder (Lembo, 1988).

*Holosystolic murmurs*
These murmurs begin with $S_1$ and extend up to and sometimes beyond $S_2$. They arise from atrio-ventricular valve regurgitation, restrictive VSDs, and some aortopulmonary connections (Perloff, 1994).

In contrast to the early systolic murmur of TR with normal right ventricular pressure, in the context of pulmonary hypertension, right ventricular pressure exceeds right atrial pressure throughout systole and hence the murmur is holosystolic. In recognition of the Mexican physician who described its characteristic increase in intensity with inspiration, it is known as Carvallo's murmur (Rivaro-Carvallo, 1946).

In mitral regurgitation, the radiation of the murmur depends on the specific pathology and direction of the resultant regurgitant jet. If a heavily fibrosed subvalvular apparatus prevents anterior leaflet coaptation, or if the posterior leaflet freely prolapses into the atrium, regurgitant flow will be directed anteriorly and medially (16). The murmur will radiate from the apex to the base of the heart. Conversely, if the jet is directed posterolaterally due to a reversal of the anatomy described above, the murmur will radiate from the apex to the axilla, scapula, or the spine where bone conduction may further radiate the murmur (Perloff and Harvey, 1962). Of course, disease of both leaflets may result in central or multiple jets producing murmurs intermediate in location.

In VSDs without pulmonary hypertension, the associated murmur is holosystolic since left ventricular pressure exceeds right ventricular pressure throughout systole. It is usually harsh and is located over the left third or fourth intercostal space, with transmission across the chest (Hollman *et al.*, 1963).

Finally, with the development of pulmonary hypertension, the continuous murmurs of aorto-pulmonary connections (e.g. aortopulmonary window or patent ductus arteriosus) become systolic as increasing pulmonary resistance limits left-to-right shunt in diastole (Nell and Mounsey, 1958).

DIASTOLIC MURMURS
These murmurs are always pathologic and hence necessitate further investigation.

*Early diastolic murmurs*
These murmurs generally arise from incompetence of the semilunar valves and exhibit considerable variation in quality and duration as a function of their chronicity. The more commonly seen chronic AR produces a high-pitched decrescendo murmur beginning with $S_2$ and lasting throughout diastole. Severe regurgitation produces a more rapidly tapering murmur since the pressure gradient separating the aorta and LV rapidly diminishes (Choudhry and Etchells, 1999).

Severe acute AR is a surgical emergency, and hence less frequently encountered. Its early diastolic murmur is shorter, ending well before $S_2$ because of the more rapid equilibration in pressure between the aorta and the nondilated, noncompliant LV. Its pitch is medium in contrast to the high pitch of chronic AR and it is usually softer (Morganroth *et al.*, 1977). Auscultation at end-exhalation improves recognition of this murmur. Radiation to the right sternal border suggests a dilated aortic root (Harvey *et al.*, 1963).

On the right side of the heart, pulmonary valve incompetence associated with pulmonary hypertension causes an early diastolic murmur known as the Graham Steell murmur. It begins with $P_2$ and persists throughout diastole. The right ventricular (RV) diastolic pressure generally remains well below PA pressure, resulting in a 'rectangular' rather than a decrescendo murmur (Perloff, 1967).

*Mid-diastolic murmurs*
These murmurs usually represent flow through stenotic atrioventricular (AV) valves, increased flow through normal valves, or pulmonary regurgitation in the absence of pulmonary hypertension.

Most common is the murmur of mitral stenosis, which is best heard at the site of the apical impulse after maneuvers to increase cardiac output (e.g. leg lifts). It is low pitched and often preceded by an opening snap (Fortuin and Craige, 1973). The length of the murmur during long pauses in atrial fibrillation provides some indication of its severity (Criley and Hermer, 1971).

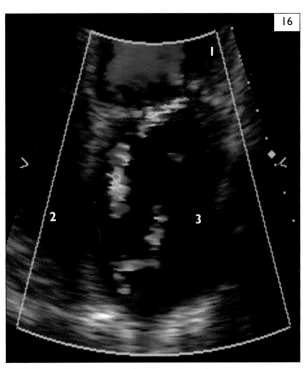

**16** Echocardiographic color flow Doppler imaging demonstrating mitral regurgitant flow directed towards the septum. 1: left ventricle; 2: right atrium; 3: left atrium.

The murmur of tricuspid stenosis is distinguished from mitral stenosis by its location at the left lower sternal border and its increase with inspiration due to the corresponding increase in RV filling (Perloff and Harvey, 1960). Increased forward flow through AV valves may also produce mid-diastolic murmurs or 'rumbles'. This occurs with severe regurgitation of either AV valve (tricuspid or mitral), an atrial septal defect (ASD) (**17–21**) with left-to-right shunt (tricuspid rumble), and a VSD with left-to-right shunt (mitral rumble).

Mid-diastolic murmurs may be heard intermittently in third degree heart block, when atrial systole occurs simultaneous with the early rapid phase of ventricular filling (Ross and Criley, 1964). Finally, a mid-diastolic murmur may occur as a result of pulmonary regurgitation in the absence of pulmonary hypertension. The more modest difference in pulmonary artery (PA) and RV pressure at the onset of diastole produces a crescendo-decrescendo murmur which begins after $P_2$.

*Late diastolic (presystolic) murmurs*
Murmurs heard in this phase of the cardiac cycle are usually produced by high velocity flow through a stenotic AV valve during atrial contraction. They often represent augmentation of a softer mid-diastolic murmur. As described above, a tricuspid origin is recognized by the murmur's prominence during inspiration and its diamond-shaped contour (Fortuin and Craige, 1973). A presystolic murmur may occur in concert with early diastolic murmur of AR. Described with a correctly predicted mechanism in the 19th century, the Austin Flint murmur is produced by the vibration of the mitral valve leaflets during atrial ejection in the face of rapidly rising LV pressure caused by aortic regurgitation (Flint, 1862).

CONTINUOUS MURMURS
This refers specifically to murmurs which continue from diastole, through $S_1$, straight on into systole. Generally, they are not produced by valvular heart disease but instead represent vascular aberrations (*Table 1*).

**Table I** Differential diagnosis of continuous thoracic murmurs in order of frequency

| Diagnosis | Key findings |
|---|---|
| Cervical venous hum | Disappears on compression of the jugular vein |
| Hepatic venous hum | Often disappears with epigastric pressure |
| Mammary soufflé | Disappears on pressing hard with stethoscope |
| Patent ductus arteriosus | Loudest at second left intercostal space |
| Coronary arteriovenous fistula | Loudest at lower sternal borders |
| Ruptured aneurysm of sinus of Valsalva | Loudest at upper right sternal border, sudden onset |
| Bronchial collaterals | Associated signs of congenital heart disease |
| | High-grade coarctation |
| | Brachial pedal arterial pressure gradient |
| Anomalous left coronary artery arising from pulmonary artery | Electrocardiographic changes of myocardial infarction |
| Pulmonary artery branch stenosis | Heard outside the area of cardiac dullness |
| Pulmonary arteriovenous fistula | Same as above |
| Atrial septal defect with mitral stenosis or atresia | Altered by the Valsalva maneuver |

(Adapted from Sapira JD (1990). *The Art and Science of Bedside Diagnosis*. Urban and Schwartzenberg, Baltimore.)

**17** Subcostal view of a patient with a sinus venosus atrial septal defect, 2D view. Note the location of the defect at the extreme base of the septum (arrow).

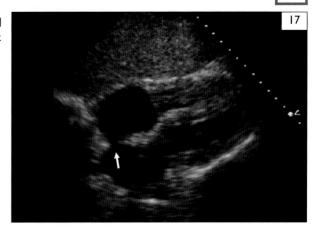

**18** Doppler color flow view of the same defect as in **17**. Note the left-to-right flow. 1: right atrium; 2: left atrium.

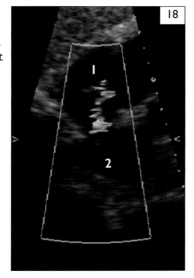

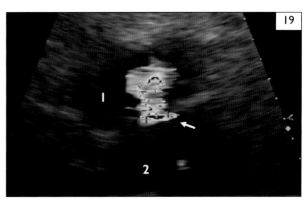

**19** Subcostal view with Doppler color flow imaging of a septum secundum atrial septal defect (arrow). Note the direction of flow from left to right. 1: right atrium; 2: left atrium.

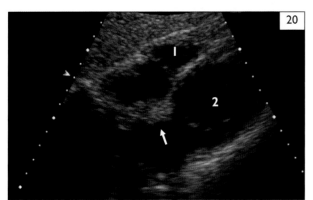

**20** Subcostal echocardiographic view of a patient who has undergone percutaneous closure of an atrial septal defect. The device accounts for the increased thickness of the interatrial septum (arrow). 1: right ventricle; 2: left ventricle.

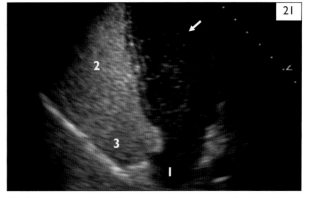

**21** Demonstration of a patent foramen ovale by apical 4-chamber imaging during injection of agitated saline and air combined with Valsalva strain. Note the microbubbles present in the left ventricle which have been shunted across the interatrial septum (arrow). 1: left atrium; 2: right ventricle; 3: right atrium.

**Further evaluation of a murmur**

The decision to pursue additional testing rests not only upon the characteristics of a murmur but also upon the degree of suspicion of valve disease prior to auscultation. Because of the limited sensitivity and specificity of physical exam, a high suspicion of valvular heart disease should not be abandoned on the basis of auscultation alone.

However, for most patients with benign histories, an algorithmic approach has been developed (22). In general, all diastolic murmurs and all continuous murmurs (with the exception of cervical venous hums or mammary souffles) should be evaluated by echocardiography. Likewise, echocardiography is indicated to evaluate systolic murmurs with the following features: (i) grade III/VI or louder; (ii) holo- or late systolic; (iii) accentuation or prolongation with Valsalva suggesting hypertrophic obstructive cardiomyopathy (HOCM) or MVP, respectively; (iv) occurring in the context of suspected endocarditis, thromboembolism, or syncope; and (v) associated with an abnormal electrocardiogram (ECG) (O'Rourke, 1998).

The American College of Cardiology and the American Heart Association (ACC/AHA) have published guidelines that outline the evidence supporting echocardiography in patients with cardiac murmurs (*Tables 2, 3*).

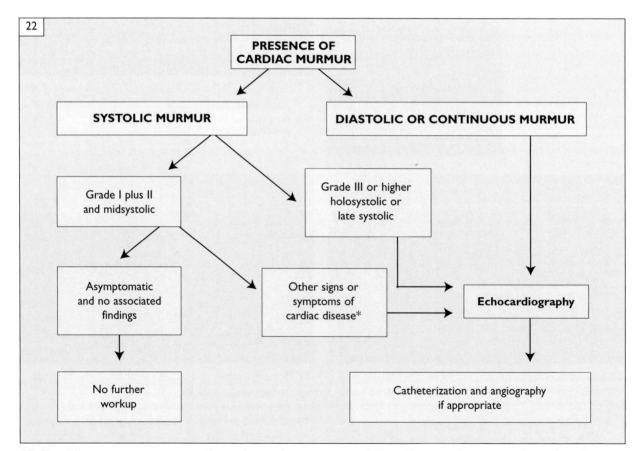

**22** Algorithm to present a strategy for evaluating heart murmurs. * If an electrocardiogram or chest X-ray has been obtained and is abnormal, an echocardiogram is recommended. (Adapted from Bonow RO, Carabello B, de Leon AC Jr, *et al.* (1998). ACC/AHA guidelines for the management of patients with valvular heart disease. *Journal of the American College of Cardiology* **32**:1486–1588, with permission.)

**Table 2** Recommendations for echocardiography in asymptomatic patients with cardiac murmurs

| Indication | Class |
|---|---|
| Diastolic or continuous murmurs | I |
| Holosystolic or late systolic murmurs | I |
| Grade III or mid systolic murmurs | I |
| Murmurs associated with abnormal physical findings on cardiac palpation or auscultation | IIa |
| Murmurs associated with abnormal ECG or chest X-ray | IIa |
| Grade II or softer midsystolic murmur identified as innocent or functional by an experienced observer | III |
| To detect 'silent' AR or MR in patients without cardiac murmurs, then recommend endocarditis prophylaxis | III |

AR: atrial regurgitation; ECG: electrocardiogram; MR: mitral regurgitation. (Adapted from Bonow RO, Carabello B, de Leon AC Jr, *et al.* (1998). ACC/AHA guidelines for the management of patients with valvular heart disease. *Journal of the American College of Cardiology* **32**:1486–1588, with permission.)

**Table 3** Recommendations for echocardiography in symptomatic patients with cardiac murmurs

| Indication | Class |
|---|---|
| Symptoms or signs of congestive heart failure, myocardial ischemia, or syncope | I |
| Symptoms or signs consistent with infective endocarditis or thromboembolism | I |
| Symptoms or signs likely due to noncardiac disease with cardiac disease not excluded by standard cardiovascular evaluation | IIa |
| Symptoms or signs of noncardiac disease with an isolated mid systolic 'innocent' murmur | III |

(Adapted from Bonow RO, Carabello B, de Leon AC Jr, *et al.* (1998). ACC/AHA guidelines for the management of patients with valvular heart disease. *Journal of the American College of Cardiology* **32**:1486–1588, with permission.)

References

Braunwald E, Perloff JK (2001). Physical examination of the heart and circulation. In: *Heart Disease: A Textbook of Cardiovascular Medicine*. E Braunwald, DP Zipes, P Libby (eds). WB Saunders, Philadelphia, pp. 48–81.

Choudhry NK, Etchells EE (1999). Does this patient have aortic regurgitation? *Journal of the American Medical Association* 281:2231–2238.

Criley JM, Hermer AJ (1971). Crescendo presystolic murmur of mitral stenosis with atrial fibrillation. *New England Journal of Medicine* 285:1284–1287.

De Leon AC, Perloff JK, Twigg H, Moyd M (1965). The straight back syndrome. *Circulation* 32:193–203.

Flint A (1862). On cardiac murmurs. *American Journal of Medical Science* 44:29–54.

Fortuin NJ, Craige E (1973). Echocardiographic studies of genesis of mitral diastolic murmurs. *British Heart Journal* 35:75–81.

Gallavardin L, Pauper-Ravault M (1925). Le soufle du retre cissement aortique peut changer de timbre et devenir musical dans se propagation apexienne. *Lyon Medicine* 523:523–529.

Harvey WP, Carrodo MA, Perloff JK (1963). 'Right sided' murmurs of aortic insufficiency. *American Journal of Medical Science* 245:533–543.

Heidenreich PA, Schnittger I, Hancock SL, Atwood JE (2004). A systolic murmur is a common presentation of aortic regurgitation detected by echocardiography. *Clinical Cardiology* 27(9):502–506.

Hollman A, Morgan JJ, Goodwin JF, *et al.* (1963). Auscultatory and phonocardiographic findings in ventricular septal defect. *Circulation* 28:94–100.

Joffe HS (1992). Genesis of Stills innocent systolic murmur. *British Heart Journal* **67**: 206.

Lembo NJ, Del'Italia LJ, Crawford MH, *et al.* (1988). Bedside diagnosis of systolic murmurs. *New England Journal of Medicine* **318**:1572–1578.

Morganroth J, Perloff JK, Zeldis SM, Dunkman WB (1977). Acute severe aortic regurgitation: pathophysiology, clinical recognition, and management. *Annals of Internal Medicine* **87**:223–232.

Nell C, Mounsey P (1958). Auscultation in patent ductus arteriosus with a description of two fistulae simulating patent ductus. *British Heart Journal* **20**:61–75.

O'Rourke R (1998) Approach to the patient with a heart murmur. In: *Primary Cardiology*. L Goldman, E Braunwald (eds). WB Saunders, Philadelphia, pp. 155–173.

Perloff JK (1967). Auscultatory and phonocardiographic manifestations of pulmonary hypertension. *Progress in Cardiovascular Disease* **9**:303–340.

Perloff JK (1994). *The Clinical Recognition of Congenital Heart Disease*, 4th edn. WB Saunders, Philadelphia.

Perloff JK, Harvey WP (1960). Clinical recognition of tricuspid stenosis. *Circulation* **22**:346–352.

Perloff JK, Harvey WP (1962). Auscultatory and phonocardiographic manifestations of pure mitral regurgitation. *Progress in Cardiovascular Disease* **5**:172–194.

Rivaro-Carvallo JM (1946). Signo para el diagnóstico de las insuficiencias tricuspideas. *Arch Inst Cardiol Mexico* **16**:531.

Ross RS, Criley JM (1964). Cineangiographic studies of the origin of cardiovascular physical signs. *Circulation* **30**:255–276.

Shaver JA (1995). Cardiac auscultation: a cost-effective diagnostic skill. *Current Problems in Cardiology* **20**:441–530.

Shry EA, Smithers MA, Mascette AM (2001). Auscultation versus echocardiography in a healthy population with precordial murmur. *American Journal of Cardiology* **87**(12):1428–1430.

# Chapter Three

# Prevention of Valvular Heart Disease

## Introduction

Before discussing the diagnosis and management of specific valve lesions, it is important to recognize the opportunities to prevent valvular heart disease. Though much of the current burden of valve disease in industrialized society is degenerative as the result of chronic inflammation, a sizable portion results from valvulopathic drugs, infections, and inadequate management of renal disease. In societies with minimal access to health care, the complications of common and easily treated infections cause the majority of valvular heart disease.

## Bacterial infective endocarditis

As outlined in greater detail in the chapter devoted to this topic, valve infections begin with a traumatized endothelial surface, usually caused by a high-speed jet stream within the heart. This may occur in congenital heart disease, severe hypertrophic cardiomyopathy, or surgically constructed shunts. Alternatively, endothelial damage may result from catheter-induced trauma or prior episodes of infective endocarditis. Platelets and fibrin are deposited on these sites of endothelial injury, resulting in non-bacterial thrombotic lesions (**23, 24**). In some patients with solid tumors, platelet and fibrin deposits appear to develop without any obvious endothelial trauma (i.e. marantic endocarditis). At this point, only a transient bacteremia is required to seed these lesions, which provide a sanctuary for bacterial growth protected from the reach of phagocytic leukocytes.

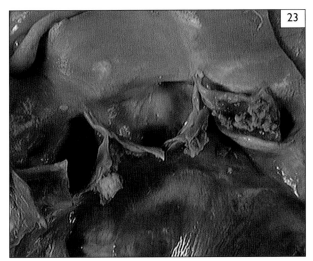

**23** Marantic vegetations on the aortic valve of an elderly female with metastatic ovarian cancer. (Courtesy of Tom Farrell, MD.)

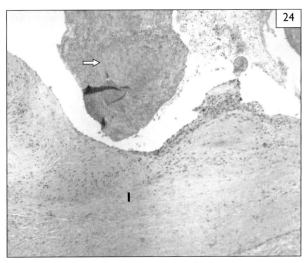

**24** Microscopic view of marantic valvular vegetations (arrow). I: valve. (Courtesy of Nora Ratcliff, MD.)

**Table 4** Recommendations for bacterial endocarditis prophylaxis

| Indication | Class |
|---|---|
| **High risk category** | I |
|   Prosthetic heart valves, including bioprosthetic homograft and allograft valves | |
|   Previous bacterial endocarditis | |
|   Complex cyanotic congenital heart disease (e.g. single ventricle states, transposition of the great arteries, tetralogy of Fallot) | |
|   Surgically constructed systemic-pulmonary shunts or conduits | |
| **Moderate risk category** | I |
|   Most other congenital cardiac malformations (other than above or below) | |
|   Acquired valvular dysfunction (e.g. rheumatic heart disease) | |
|   Hypertrophic cardiomyopathy | |
|   MVP with auscultatory evidence of valvular regurgitation and/or thickened leaflets | |
| **Low- or negligible risk category** | III |
|   Isolated secundum atrial septal defect | |
|   Surgical repair of atrial septal defect, ventricular septal defect, or patent ductus arteriosus (without residua >6 months) | |
|   Previous coronary artery bypass graft surgery | |
|   MVP without valvular regurgitation | |
|   Physiological, functional, or innocent heart murmurs | |
|   Previous Kawasaki disease without valvular dysfunction | |
|   Cardiac pacemakers and implanted defibrillators | |

MVP: mitral valve prolapse. (Adapted from Dajani AS, Taubert KA, Wilson W, *et al.* (1997). Prevention of bacterial endocarditis: recommendations by the American Heart Association. *Circulation* **96**:358–366.)

**Table 5** Endocarditis prophylaxis for dental procedures

| Endocarditis prophylaxis recommended | Endocarditis prophylaxis not recommended |
|---|---|
| **Dental extractions** | Restorative dentistry[†] (operative and prosthodontic) with/without retraction cord |
| Periodontal procedures, including surgery, scaling and root planing, probing, recall maintenance | Local anesthetic injections (nonintraligamentary)[*] |
| Dental implant placement and reimplantation of avulsed teeth | Intracanal endodontic treatment: postplacement and buildup |
| Endodontic (root canal) instrumentation of surgery only beyond the apex | Placement of rubber dams |
| Subgingival placement of antibiotic fibers/strips | Postoperative suture removal |
| Initial placement of orthodontic bands but not brackets | Placement of removable prosthodontic/orthodontic appliances |
| Intraligamentary local anesthetic injections[*] | Taking of oral impressions |
| Prophylactic cleaning of teeth or implants where bleeding is anticipated | Fluoride treatments |
| | Taking of oral radiographs |
| | Orthodontic appliance adjustment |
| | Shedding of primary teeth |

[*]Intraligamentary injections are directed between the root and bone to deliver anesthetic agents to the periosteum of the bone. [†]Includes filling cavities and replacement of missing teeth. In selected circumstances, especially with significant bleeding, antibiotic use may be indicated. (Adapted from Bonow RO, Carabello B, de Leon AC Jr, *et al.* (1998). ACC/AHA guidelines for the management of patients with valvular heart disease: a report of the American College of Cardiology/American Heart Association Task Force on Practice Guidelines (Committee on Management of Patients with Valvular Heart Disease). *Journal of the American College of Cardiology* **32**:1486–1588.)

While many instances of bacteremia are unpredictable (e.g. pneumonia), some are iatrogenic. The latter result from procedures which involve significant trauma to a colonized or infected site (e.g. dental, gastrointestinal [GI], or genitourinary [GU] procedures). On the basis of animal studies, the American Heart Association (AHA) has made recommendations regarding the prevention of endocarditis (Dajani *et al.*, 1997). Prophylaxis is recommended for cardiac conditions considered at moderate or high risk (*Table 4*). Likewise, medical and dental procedures are stratified to those which do and do not require antibiotics (*Tables 5, 6*). To address the variation in flora residing in the mouth,

---

**Table 6** Endocarditis prophylaxis for nondental procedures

**Endocarditis prophylaxis recommended**

Respiratory tract
  Tonsillectomy/adenoidectomy
  Surgical operations involving respiratory mucosa
  Bronchoscopy with rigid bronchoscope
Gastrointestinal tract (prophylaxis for high-risk
  patients; optimal for moderate risk)
  Sclerotherapy for esophageal varices
  Esophageal stricture dilation
  Endoscopic retrograde cholangiography with biliary
    obstruction
  Biliary tract surgery
  Surgical operations involving intestinal mucosa
Genitourinary tract
  Prostatic surgery
  Cystoscopy
  Urethral dilation

**Endocarditis prophylaxis not recommended**

Respiratory tract
  Endotracheal intubation
  Bronchoscopy with a flexible bronchoscope, with
    or without biopsy*
  Tympanostomy tube insertion

Gastrointestinal tract
  Transesophageal echocardiography*
  Endoscopy with or without gastrointestinal biopsy*
Genitourinary tract
  Vaginal hysterectomy*
  Vaginal delivery*
  Cesarian section
    In uninfected tissue:
    Urethral catheterization
    Uterine dilation and curettage
    Therapeutic abortion
    Sterilization procedures
    Insertion or removal of intrauterine devices

**Other**

Cardiac catheterization, including balloon angioplasty
Implantation of cardiac pacemakers, implantable
  defibrillators, and coronary stents
Incision or biopsy of surgically scrubbed skin
Circumcision

*Prophylaxis is optional for high-risk patients. (Adapted from Bonow RO, Carabello B, de Leon AC Jr, *et al.* (1998). ACC/AHA guidelines for the management of patients with valvular heart disease: a report of the American College of Cardiology/American Heart Association Task Force on Practice Guidelines (Committee on Management of Patients with Valvular Heart Disease). *Journal of the American College of Cardiology* **32**:1486–1588.)

lower GI, and GU tracts, the choice of antibiotics is tailored to address the resident flora of the body cavity, the level of risk to the patient, and any adverse drug reaction history (*Tables 7, 8*).

## Rheumatic fever prophylaxis

In comparison to incidence rates early in the twentieth century, rheumatic fever is now uncommon in populations with access to health care. However, recent epidemiologic studies suggest there has been a resurgence of rheumatic fever, beginning in 1987 (Ryan *et al.*, 2000). The damaging valvulitis is believed to result from the immunologic reaction associated with M protein serotypes of Group A streptococci. Hence, primary prevention of rheumatic fever hinges upon the accurate and timely recognition of Group A streptococcal infections. Point-of-care test kits with specificity exceeding 95% facilitate this but should be backed up by culture because of the kits' limited sensitivity (Johansson and Mansson, 2003). A previous episode of rheumatic fever predisposes to recurrent episodes, each one potentially causing further valvular damage. For this reason, continual antibiotic administration (secondary prevention) is indicated as outlined in *Table 9* (Dajani *et al.*, 1995). The prevention, diagnosis, and management of rheumatic fever was recently reviewed in a practical report published by the World Health Organization (2004.)

**Table 7** Endocarditis prophylaxis regimens for dental, oral, respiratory tract, or esophageal procedures

| Situation | Agent | Regimen* |
|---|---|---|
| Standard general prophylaxis | Amoxicillin | Adults: 2.0 g; children: 50 mg/kg PO 1 hour before procedure |
| Unable to take oral medication | Ampicillin | Adults: 2.0 g IM or IV; children: medication 50 mg/kg IM or IV within 30 minutes before procedure |
| Penicillin-allergic | Clindamycin or cephalexin* | Adults: 600 mg; children: 20 mg/kg PO 1 hour before procedure |
| | or cephadroxil† | Adults: 2.0 g; children: 50 mg/kg PO 1 hour before procedure |
| | or azithromycin or clarithromycin | Adults 500 mg; children: 15 mg/kg PO 1 hour before procedure |
| Penicillin-allergic and unable to take oral medications | Clindamycin | Adults: 600 mg; children: 20 mg/kg IV within 30 minutes before procedure |
| | or cefazolin† | Adults: 1.0 g; children: 25 mg/kg IMor IV within 30 minutes before procedure |

*Total children's dose should not exceed adult dose. †Cephalosporins should not be used in individuals with immediate-type hypersensitivity reaction (urticaria, angioedema, or anaphylaxis) to penicillins. (Adapted from Bonow RO, Carabello B, de Leon AC Jr, et al. (1998). ACC/AHA guidelines for the management of patients with valvular heart disease: a report of the American College of Cardiology/American Heart Association Task Force on Practice Guidelines (Committee on Management of Patients with Valvular Heart Disease). *Journal of the American College of Cardiology* **32**:1486–1588.)

**Table 8** Endocarditis prophylaxis regimens for genitourinary, gastrointestinal (excluding esophageal) procedures

| Situation | Agent(s)* | Regimens[†] |
|---|---|---|
| High-risk patients | Ampicillin plus gentamicin | Adults: ampicillin 2.0 g IM/IV plus gentamicin 1.5 mg/kg (not to exceed 120 mg) within 30 minutes of starting the procedure. Six hours later, ampicillin 1 g IM/IV or amoxicillin 1 g PO. Children: ampicillin 50 mg/kg IM or IV (not to exceed 2.0 g) plus gentamicin1.5 mg/kg within 30 minutes of starting procedure. Six hours later, ampicillin 25mg/kg IM/IV or amoxicillin 25mg/kg PO. |
| High-risk patients allergic to ampicillin/amoxicillin | Vancomycin plus gentamicin | Adults: vancomycin 1.0 g IV over 1–2 hours plus gentamicin 1.5 mg/kg IV/IM (not to exceed 120 mg). Complete injection/infusion within 30 minutes of starting the procedure. Children: vancomycin 20 mg/kg IV over 1–2 hours plus gentamicin 1.5 mg/kg IV/IM. Complete injection/infusion within 30 minutes of starting the procedure. |
| Moderate-risk patients | Amoxicillin or ampicillin | Adults: amoxicillin 2.0 g PO 1 hour before procedure, or ampicillin 2.0 g IM/IV within 30 minutes of starting the procedure. Children: amoxicillin 50 mg/kg PO 1 hour before procedure, or ampicillin 50 mg/kg IM/IV within 30 minutes of starting the procedure |
| Moderate-risk patients allergic to ampicillin/amoxicillin | Vancomycin | Adults: vancomycin 1.0 g IV over 1–2 hours. Complete infusion within 30 minutes of starting the procedure. Children: vancomycin 20mg/kg over 1–2 hours. Complete infusion within 30 minutes of starting the procedure. |

* No second dose of vancomycin or gentamicin is recommended. [†] Total children's dose should not exceed adult dose. (Adapted from Bonow RO, Carabello B, de Leon AC Jr, *et al.* (1998). ACC/AHA guidelines for the management of patients with valvular heart disease: a report of the American College of Cardiology/American Heart Association Task Force on Practice Guidelines (Committee on Management of Patients with Valvular Heart Disease). *Journal of the American College of Cardiology* **32**:1486–1588.)

**Table 9** Secondary prevention of rheumatic fever

| Agent | Dose | Mode |
|---|---|---|
| Benzathine | 1,200,000 U every 4 weeks | IM |
| Penicillin G | (every 3 weeks for high-risk* patients such as those with residual carditis) | |
| Penicillin V | 250 mg twice daily or | Oral |
| Sulfadiazine | 0.5 g once daily for patients <27 kg (60 lb) 1.0 g once daily for patients >27 kg (60 lb) | Oral |
| For individuals allergic to penicillin and sulfadiazine | | |
| Erythromycin | 250 mg twice daily | Oral |

*High–risk patients include patients with residual rheumatic carditis as well as patients from economically disadvantaged populations. (Adapted from Bonow RO, Carabello B, de Leon AC Jr, *et al.* (1998). ACC/AHA guidelines for the management of patients with valvular heart disease: a report of the American College of Cardiology/American Heart Association Task Force on Practice Guidelines (Committee on Management of Patients with Valvular Heart Disease). *Journal of the American College of Cardiology* **32**:1486–1588.)

## Metabolic disorders

Until recently, the calcification of the aortic annulus, valve, and arch was believed to represent a passive degenerative process related to aging. However, it is now recognized that both biomechanical and metabolic abnormalities contribute to the development of valvular calcification. In particular, diabetes, hypercholesterolemia, and end-stage renal disease (ESRD) are all risk factors. Hence, meticulous blood sugar and lipid management are essential. In the case of renal disease, dystrophic calcification may be discouraged by maintaining a calcium-phosphorus product below 70 $mg^2/dl^2$. Since the calcification results primarily from elevations in phosphorus, key measures include: (i) limiting dietary intake; (ii) use of calcium-free phosphate binders; and (iii) cautious lowering of dialysate calcium concentration (London et al., 2000).

## Valvulopathic agents

There is limited understanding of agents thought to be deleterious to cardiac valves. Best known are the anoretic drugs. Reports in 1997 appeared to link left-sided regurgitant valve lesions with diet drugs; consequently, fenfluramine, phenteramine, and dexfenfluramine were taken off the US market. In light of these experiences, a cautious approach should be taken to the use of any future anoretic agent involving the serotonin pathway.

## References

Anonymous (2004). Rheumatic fever and rheumatic heart disease. *World Health Organization Technical Report Series* **923**:1–122, back cover.

Bonow RO, Carabello B, de Leon AC Jr, *et al.* (1998). ACC/AHA guidelines for the management of patients with valvular heart disease: a report of the American College of Cardiology/American Heart Association Task Force on Practice Guidelines (Committee on Management of Patients with Valvular Heart Disease). *Journal of the American College of Cardiology* **32**:1486–1588.

Dajani A, Taubert K, Ferrieri P, Peter G, Shulman S (1995). Treatment of acute streptococcal pharyngitis and prevention of rheumatic fever: a statement for health professionals: Committee on Rheumatic Fever, Endocarditis, and Kawasaki Disease of the Council on Cardiovascular Disease in the Young, The American Heart Association. *Pediatrics* **96**:758–764.

Dajani AS, Taubert KA, Wilson W, *et al.* (1997). Prevention of bacterial endocarditis: recommendations by the American Heart Association. *Circulation* **96**:358–366.

Johansson L, Mansson NO (2003). Rapid test, throat culture, and clinical assessment in the diagnosis of tonsillitis. *Family Practice* **20**(2):108–111.

London GM, Pannier B, Marchais SJ, Guerin AP (2000). Calcification of the aortic valve in the dialyzed patient. *Journal of the American Society of Nephrology* **11**(4):778–783.

Ryan M, Antony JH, Grattan-Smith PJ (2000). Sydenham's Chorea: a resurgence in the 1990s? *Journal of Pediatrics and Child Health* **36**(1):95–96.

# Chapter Four

# Aortic Stenosis

## Definition

Aortic stenosis (AS) refers to congenital or acquired obstruction of blood flow through the aortic valve. However, in addition, some authors use the term in reference to supra- and subvalvular pathology. Supravalvular aortic stenosis is a rare form of outflow obstruction. The narrowing may be discreet or long and tubular. It is a congenital defect associated with elfin faces, hypercalcemia, mental retardation, and peripheral pulmonic stenosis (William's Syndrome). Subvalvular stenosis may be caused by a ridge extending into the outflow tract, a cylindrical constriction of the outflow tract or, in hypertrophic cardiomyopathy, by obstruction caused by the anterior movement of the mitral valve leaflets. In some patients this is present only at diminished left ventricular (LV) volumes recreated in the echocardiography laboratory by Valsalva (25–27). The turbulent flow produced may damage the aortic valve and subsequently cause aortic regurgitation (Nishimura, 2000).

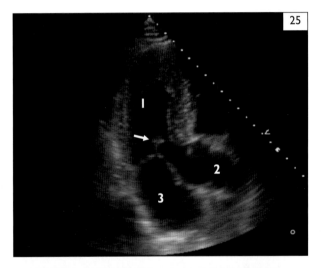

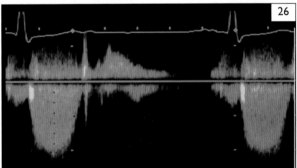

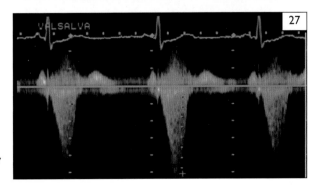

**25–27** Multiple views of a patient with a dynamic left ventricular outflow tract (LVOT) obstruction.
**25** Apical 3-chamber view demonstrating systolic anterior motion of the closed mitral valve leaflets (arrow) drawn towards the interventricular septum, by the Venturi effect of high velocity flow through the narrowed outflow tract. 1: left ventricle; 2: ascending aorta; 3: left atrium.
**26** Continuous wave Doppler interrogation of the same patient from the apex through the LVOT and aortic valve, demonstrating a modestly elevated velocity of 2 m/s.
**27** Repeat continuous wave interrogation with Valsalva, demonstrating dynamic obstruction with an increase in velocity to 5 m/s and a characteristic dagger-shaped flow envelope (scimitar sign).

## Etiology

In children and young adults, congenital malformation is the most common etiology. In order of descending prevalence, the valve malformations are bicuspid, unicuspid, indeterminate, and hypoplastic (28, 29). Interestingly, aortic coarctation is over-represented in patients with anomalous aortic valves (30–32).

Older patients are more likely to have acquired aortic valve stenosis. In industrialized societies, a fibrocalcific process underlies most cases (33, 34). The pathogenesis appears similar to atherosclerosis with risk factors of age, diabetes mellitus, hypertension, hyperlipidemia, and histologic features of inflammation (Otto *et al.*, 1994). Paralleling the controversy in coronary artery disease, some evidence suggests that Chlamydia infection may play a role (Juvonen *et al.*, 1998). Rheumatic heart disease causes a distinctive pattern of calcification which begins with tiny nodules along the lines of valve closure. This is followed by fibrin deposition on the cusps and loss of normal valve morphology. Over decades, this process may result in fusion of the commisures, calcification of the cusps, and fibrosis of the chordae (Neithardt and Sorrentino, 2003). However, it rarely affects the aortic valve alone and, while common in developing societies, it is increasingly rare in western society. Paget's disease of the bone and end-stage renal disease are rare causes of aortic stenosis.

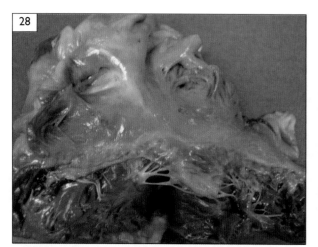

**28** Pathologic specimen of a normal aortic valve. (Courtesy of Nora Ratcliff, MD.)

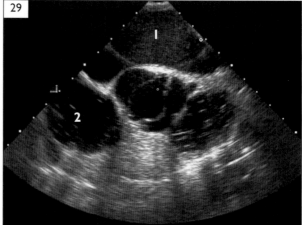

**29** Parasternal short axis echocardiographic view at the base of the heart of a patient with a bicuspid aortic valve (valve seen en face in the center of the picture). 1: right outflow tract; 2: right atrium.

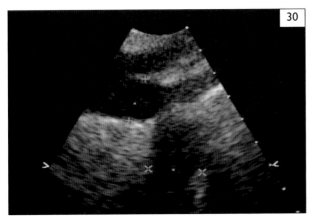

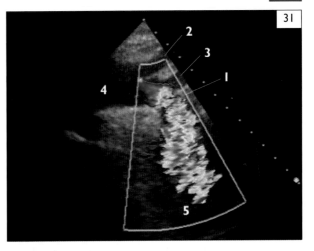

**30–32** Multiple views of a patient with coarctation of the aorta, an anomaly associated with bicuspid aortic valves. **30** 2D view of the transverse aorta seen in longitudinal view, demonstrating the coarctation lying just distal to the left subclavian artery and the presence of poststenotic dilatation. **31** Doppler color flow view demonstrating high velocity and turbulent flow distal to the coarctation (1). 2: left common carotid; 3: left subclavian; 4: ascending aorta; 5: descending aorta. **32** Continuous wave Doppler interrogation documenting peak instantaneous gradients varying from 22–39 mmHg (2.9–5.2 kPa). The variation is due to the irregular rhythm and inconsistent filling of the left ventricle.

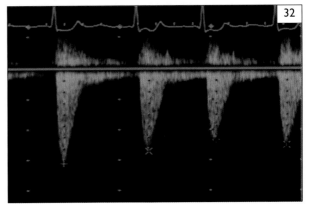

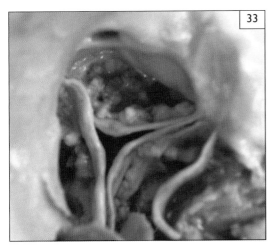

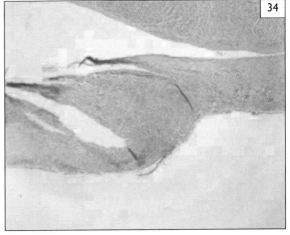

**33** An aortic valve with heavy calcification of the cusps. Note that the valve edges are spared. (Courtesy of Tom Farrell, MD.)

**34** Microscopic view of a thickened, scarred valve leaflet. (Courtesy of Nora Ratcliff, MD.)

## Pathophysiology

The cross-sectional area of a normal aortic valve is 3–4 cm$^2$. While reductions in valve area to 1.5–2.0 cm$^2$ cause a minimal pressure gradient, further narrowing produces dramatic increases in the mean pressure gradient (*Table 10*) (Carabello, 2002).

Obstruction to flow usually develops slowly, thereby allowing the LV to adapt by thickening (*35*). This concentric hypertrophy serves to reduce wall stress (the law of Laplace describes wall tension as directly proportional to pressure and radius and inversely proportional to thickness). As long as the process of muscular wall thickening keeps pace with narrowing of the aortic orifice, the wall tension is maintained. This homeostasis comes at a price, however. The thickened walls are less compliant, rendering the ventricle less able to fill rapidly. Achievement of adequate end-diastolic volume becomes heavily dependent upon atrial contraction. This diastolic dysfunction is dramatically exposed by the onset of atrial fibrillation, which often precipitates acute congestive heart failure (CHF) in patients with severe AS.

Another consequence of the concentric hypertrophy is increased myocardial oxygen demand. When coupled with reduced coronary flow due to an abbreviated diastole and low diastolic pressures, this hypertrophy predisposes to subendocardial ischemia, even in the presence of normal coronary arteries. Ventricular arrhythmias are more common as well. Finally, exertional syncope may develop as exercise-induced peripheral vasodilation occurs in the context of a fixed cardiac output. The resulting decrease in blood pressure may reduce cerebral perfusion below the minimum required for consciousness.

## Clinical presentation

### SYMPTOMS

Patients with mild or moderate AS are usually asymptomatic unless they have coexisting cardiopulmonary disease or infective endocarditis intervenes. Even patients with severe stenosis often remain asymptomatic until the ventricle begins to fail. At this point, they usually develop fatigue followed by the cardinal symptoms of angina, syncope, and dyspnea. Average survival following the onset of these symptoms is 2 years, 3 years, and 5 years, respectively (Ross and Braunwald, 1968). In rare instances, sudden death is the tragic, first manifestation of disease.

**Table 10** Relation of the aortic valve area to the mean gradient*

| Aortic valve area (cm$^2$) | Mean gradient (mmHg/kPa) |
|---|---|
| 4 | 1.7/0.2 |
| 3 | 2.9/0.4 |
| 2 | 6.6/0.9 |
| 1 | 26/3.5 |
| 0.9 | 32/4.3 |
| 0.8 | 41/5.5 |
| 0.7 | 53/7.1 |
| 0.6 | 73/9.7 |
| 0.5 | 105/14 |

\* Data were derived with the Gorlin formula: aortic valve area = [CO × 1000]/[44.3 × SEP × HR] × √ mean pressure gradient, where the cardiac output (CO) was assumed to be 6 l/min, the systolic ejection period (SEP) was assumed to be 0.33 sec, and the heart rate (HR) was assumed to be 80 beats per minute. (Adapted from Carabello BA (2002). Aortic stenosis. *New England Journal of Medicine* **346**(9):677–682, with permission. Copyright Massachusetts Medical Society. All rights reserved.)

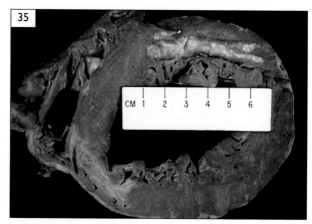

**35** Pathologic specimen of severe left ventricular hypertrophy (note the thickness of the free wall) and multiple infarcts in a patient who had severe aortic stenosis and coronary atherosclerosis which often accompanies it. (Courtesy of Tom Farrell, MD.)

In sedentary patients, it may be unclear whether they are inactive by choice or have gradually curtailed their activity due to symptoms. In these cases, performing a treadmill stress test with close physician supervision may be helpful. As an operational definition of 'asymptomatic', the European Society of Cardiology (ESC) Working Group on Valvular Heart Disease suggests the ability to reach 80% of predicted maximal heart rate without symptoms (Iung *et al.*, 2002).

SIGNS

The classic finding in the assessment of peripheral pulses is a delayed and slowly rising wave contour (pulsus parvus et tardus). However, it may be absent in patients with associated aortic regurgitation or calcified, inelastic arteries. In the carotids, a shudder produced by systolic vibrations may be palpable. Prominent jugular a waves may be seen as a result of septal hypertrophy and its attendant decrease in right ventricular (RV) compliance. In advanced disease, LV failure leads to pulmonary hypertension, RV failure, and tricuspid regurgitation. In this instance, giant v waves will be evident upon inspection of the neck.

Precordial palpation may reveal a sustained and inferolaterally displaced cardiac impulse. Because the hypertrophied LV is noncompliant, the important contribution to filling provided by atrial contraction may be evident as a palpable $S_4$. In severe AS, a systolic thrill is often palpable at the base of the heart.

Auscultation reveals a variety of abnormal heart sounds as the LV fails. $S_1$ becomes soft because of the diminished force of LV contraction. With decreasing valve mobility, $S_2$ may disappear as $A_2$ decreases in intensity due to diminished valve excursion and $P_2$ becomes obscured by the systolic murmur. However, if the underlying etiology is congenital bicuspid AS, the flexible leaflets may produce both an aortic ejection sound by their abrupt cessation of opening (approximately 60 msec after $S_1$) and a prominent $A_2$ due to their snappy closure (Braunwald, 2001).

The murmur of AS was discussed in Chapter 2. Of special note, patients with aortic sclerosis but no significant obstruction generally have softer, more musical murmurs (Otto, 1999). In addition, many patients with AS also have aortic regurgitation (AR) manifest by its characteristic high-pitched, decrescendo murmur. In the last stages of progressive AS, pump function becomes so impaired that the murmur often decreases in intensity (**36**).

**36** Severe calcific aortic stenosis in a 56-year-old female. The systolic ejection murmur is prolonged and midpeaking. The soft $S_2$ suggests immobility of the aortic cusps. Note the slow carotid upstroke. AA: aortic area; DM: diastolic murmur; SM: systolic murmur. (Adapted from Tavel ME (1972). *Clinical Phonocardiography and External Pulse Recording.* Yearbook Medical Publishers, Chicago.)

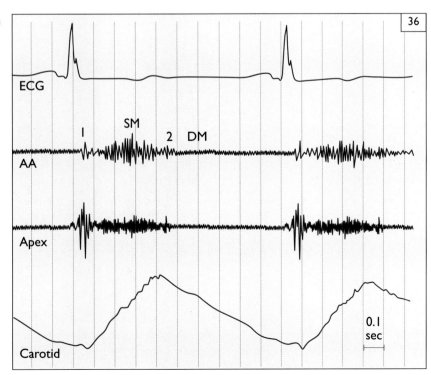

LABORATORY FINDINGS

*Electrocardiography*

Common features on the electrocardiogram include left ventricular hypertrophy (LVH) with a strain pattern and a biphasic p wave in $V_1$ corresponding to left atrial (LA) hypertrophy. Atrioventricular and intraventricular conduction abnormalities may be seen when calcification extends from the valve into the conduction system (37).

*Chest radiography*

On the chest X-ray rounding of the left heart border and apex, post stenotic dilation of the aorta, calcification of the aortic valve, and pulmonary venous congestion may be apparent. Note, however, that these findings are neither highly sensitive nor specific (38, 39).

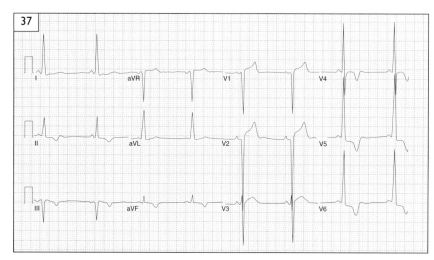

**37** 12-lead electrocardiogram demonstrating findings of left ventricular hypertrophy with repolarization abnormalities consistent with 'strain'. (Courtesy of Frances DeRook, MD.)

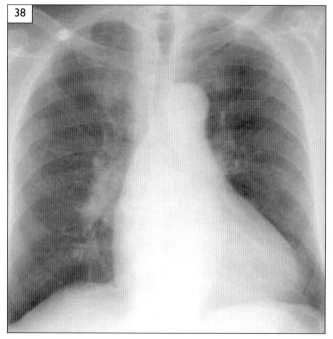
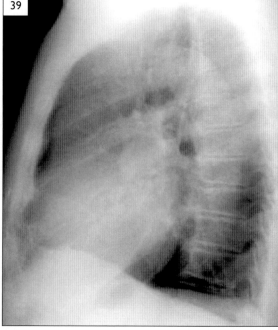

**38, 39** Postero-anterior and lateral chest films of a patient with severe aortic stenosis and aortic insufficiency. Note the increase in cardiothoracic ratio and the vascular prominence and peribronchial cuffing, suggestive of pulmonary venous hypertension. (Courtesy of Bill Black, MD.)

## *Echocardiography*

Echocardiography serves as the principal modality for confirming and quantitating AS. 2D imaging (**40**) provides information on chamber size, degree of hypertrophy, LV systolic function, valve mobility, and calcification (Okura, 1997). Doppler measurement of transvalvular blood flow velocity can be used to determine peak and mean pressure gradients using the modified Bernoulli equation $[P = 4v^2]$ (Leborgne *et al.*, 1998). The aortic valve area may also be estimated using echocardiographically obtained data (*Table 11*). In patients with a low cardiac output and aortic stenosis, the velocity of blood flow through the valve may not be dramatically elevated despite severe stenosis. Repeating the echocardiographic assessment of aortic valve area after raising the cardiac output by 30% with IV dobutamine may distinguish valve immobility caused by poor LV systolic function from that caused by true 'fixed' aortic stenosis (Monin *et al.*, 2003).

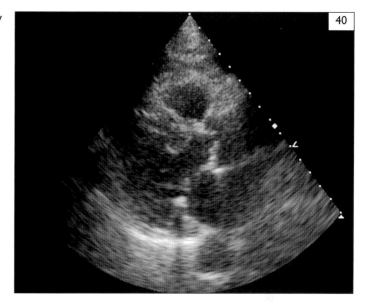

**40** Parasternal long axis echocardiographic view of the heart. Note the limited opening of the aortic valve and calcification evidenced by the bright echo reflections.

**Table 11** Calculation of peak and mean aortic pressure gradients and estimated aortic valve area from echocardiographic data

| | Measure used | Selected measure | 1 | 2 | 3 | 4 | 5 |
|---|---|---|---|---|---|---|---|
| Ao V$_2$ max | 318 cm/sec | avg | 323 | 311 | 315 | 317 | 323 |
| Ao V$_2$ trace | 23.6 | avg | 24.2 | 22.5 | 24.1 | 23.3 | 23.6 |
| Ao V$_2$ VTI | 67.1 cm | avg | 70.2 | 68.0 | 67.9 | 64.4 | 65.0 |
| LV V$_1$ max | 103 cm/sec | avg | 103 | 104 | 100 | 103 | 104 |
| LV V$_1$ trace | 2.79 | avg | 2.69 | 2.75 | 2.68 | 2.86 | 2.95 |
| LV V$_1$ VTI | 22.9 cm | avg | 20.4 | 23.5 | 23.3 | 23.7 | 23.4 |
| LVOT diam | 1.94 cm | avg | 1.93 | 1.94 | | | |
| Ao max PG | 40.4 mmHg (5.4 kPa) | AO max PG2 | | 36.2 mmHg (4.8 kPa) | | | |
| Ao mean PG | 23.6 mmHg (3.2 kPa) | AO mean PG2 | | 20.8 mmHg (2.8 kPa) | | | |
| AVA (VD) | 0.951 cm$^2$ | AVA (ID) | | 1.00 cm$^2$ | | | |

Ao: aorta; AVA: aortic valve area; ID: integral-derived; LV: left ventricle; LVOT: left ventricular outflow tract; PG: pressure gradient; V: velocity; VD: velocity-derived; VTI: velocity time integral.

*Cardiac catheterization*

Historically, invasive hemodynamic assessment has been the gold standard for quantitating AS. Currently, it continues to serve an important role in patients with technically poor ultrasound windows and in cases when clinical and echocardiographic information conflict. Simultaneous pressure measurements within the LV and in the ascending aorta (**41**) combined with cardiac output (CO) established by thermodilution or the Fick method allow calculation of the aortic valve area (AVA) by the Gorlin equation [AVA = CO × 1000/(44.3 × SEP × HR × √pressure gradient)] where HR = heart rate, and SEP = systolic ejection period. Left ventriculography may be hazardous in the presence of an elevated LV end-diastolic pressure (LVEDP) and hence is often omitted. Even without left ventriculography, the simple act of attempting to pass a wire across a highly calcified and stenotic valve poses risk of embolization. This has been established by serial cerebral magnetic resonance imaging (MRI) studies (Meine and Harrison, 2004). For this reason, the practice of routinely determining AVA by invasive means is controversial (Chambers *et al.*, 2004). In patients with any coronary artery disease (CAD) risk factors, coronary angiography is commonly performed prior to valve surgery to assess the need for concomitant bypass surgery.

*Cardiac magnetic resonance*

With more powerful magnets, faster computers, and innovative software cardiac magnetic resonance (CMR) is playing an increasingly important role in the evaluation of AS. While velocity encoded imaging is now beginning to provide hemodynamic assessments, the best established role of CMR is in determining AVA by planimetry (Kupfahl *et al.*, 2004).

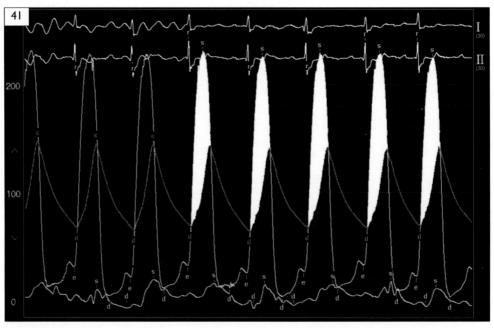

**41** Simultaneous pressure tracings from the aorta (purple, AO), left ventricle (yellow, LV), and pulmonary artery (blue). Note the large systolic pressure gradient separating the LV and AO.

## Treatment

### MEDICAL MANAGEMENT

Patient education is critical. Patients with asymptomatic severe AS must understand the need to seek attention if they develop the cardinal symptoms mentioned earlier, and the need for infective endocarditis prophylaxis. In addition, they should avoid strenuous activity. As noted above, closely supervised treadmill exercise electrocardiogram (ECG) may be employed in sedentary patients to identify those with unrecognized severe limitations. The European Society of Cardiology working group has suggested the following criteria for considering the test as positive: symptoms of dyspnea, angina, syncope or near syncope; failure to raise systolic blood pressure by 20 mmHg (2.7 kPa); inability to reach 80% of predicted maximal heart rate, >2 mm horizontal or down sloping ST segment depression in comparison to resting ST segment position in the absence of other explanations, ventricular tachycardia (Iung *et al.*, 2002).

Since the rate of progression ranges from 0–0.3 cm² per year and is unpredictable for an individual patient, serial echocardiography is indicated. Evidence suggests that patients with fibrocalcific disease progress faster than those with bicuspid or rheumatic disease (Iung *et al.*, 2002). In some studies, CAD, increasing age, hypertension, smoking, and hyperlipidemia have been identified as predictors of rapid progression (Peter *et al.*, 1993). Biannual evaluations are reasonable in mild disease, but annual or semiannual evaluations are recommended in severe disease. A recent prospective study of consecutive patients has suggested that patients with an increase in peak velocity exceeding 0.3 m/sec per year have a greatly increased likelihood of requiring aortic valve replacement (AVR) (Rosenhek *et al.*, 2000). Epidemiologic evidence suggests that hydroxymethylglutaryl coenzyme A (HMG-CoA) reductase inhibitors may slow the rate of valve stenosis (Novaro *et al.*, 2001).

Once patients become symptomatic, medical therapy becomes subordinate to surgical intervention (**42**). In patients unable or unwilling to undergo surgery, digoxin may be helpful if the LV ejection fraction (LVEF) is diminished, but carries a small risk of arrhythmias. Diuretics and nitrates should be used cautiously to avoid decompensation from inadequate preload. Beta-blockers are usually avoided because of their negative inotropic effect. Atrial fibrillation should prompt an attempt to restore sinus rhythm, usually by direct current cardioversion. Coexisting mitral valve disease should be excluded by physical exam and echocardiography.

**42** Survival among patients with severe symptomatic aortic stenosis who underwent valve replacement and similar patients who declined to undergo surgery. Closed circles: valve replacement; open circles: no surgery. (Adapted from Schwartz F, Baumann P, Manthey J, *et al.* (1982). The effect of aortic valve replacement on survival. *Circulation* **66**:1105–1110.)

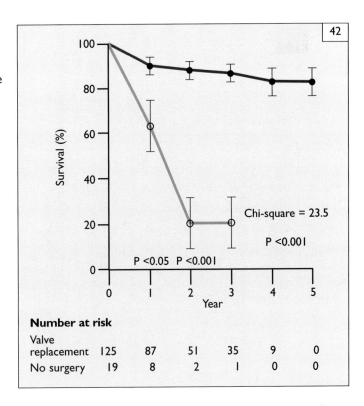

## Percutaneous intervention

Aortic balloon valvotomy, performed by inflating a balloon placed across the valve, is often very effective in adolescents and young adults with congenital AS, but in adults with calcific AS, the procedure's approximate 10% complication rate and frequent restenosis renders it a poor substitute for AVR (Lieberman *et al.*, 1995). However, it may serve as a bridge to definitive surgical therapy by allowing hemodynamic stabilization of a critically ill patient (*Table 12*). Aortic balloon valvotomy is never indicated in asymptomatic individuals, due to the risk and its limited efficacy.

One of the most exciting therapeutic developments in valvular heart disease is the development of an aortic valve which could be implanted percutaneously. Its first use in a patient has occurred with favorable short-term hemodynamic results (Cribier *et al.*, 2003). Though not yet ready for widespread implementation, the approach holds promise.

## Surgical intervention

In calcific aortic stenosis, valve repair is very rarely possible (**43**). AVR is indicated in symptomatic patients with AVA <0.9 cm$^2$ or AVA index <0.6 cm$^2$/m$^2$ of body surface area. US guidelines suggest that symptomatic patients be considered for surgery (*Table 13*) in the presence of progressive LV dysfunction, a hypotensive response to exercise, and at the time of bypass surgery. European guidelines include these indications as well as the presence of moderate to severe calcification, with a peak aortic velocity >4 m/sec and an annual interval increase in velocity of 0.3 m/sec; severe LVH with >15 mm wall thickness in the absence of hypertension, and severe otherwise unexplained ventricular arrhythmias (Iung *et al.*, 2002).

The operative (30-day) mortality in a recent national database of 26,317 patients was 4.3% (Jamieson *et al.*, 1999). However, this varies with surgical skill, post operative care, and patient factors. Some surgeons utilize a transverse sternotomy, described as minimally invasive surgery, in the interest of reducing post operative discomfort. No randomized trial of this approach has been performed.

---

**Table 12** Recommendations for aortic balloon valvotomy in adults with aortic stenosis*

| Indication | Class |
|---|---|
| A 'bridge' to surgery in hemodynamically unstable patients who are at high risk for AVR | IIa |
| Palliation in patients with serious comorbid conditions | IIb |
| Patients who require urgent noncardiac surgery | IIb |
| An alternative to AVR | III |

* Recommendations for aortic balloon valvotomy in adolescents and young adults with aortic stenosis are provided in section VI.A. of these guidelines. AVR: aortic valve replacement. (Adapted from Bonow RO, Carabello B, de Leon AC Jr, et al. (1998). ACC/AHA guidelines for the management of patients with valvular heart disease. *Journal of the American College of Cardiology* **32**:1486–1588.)

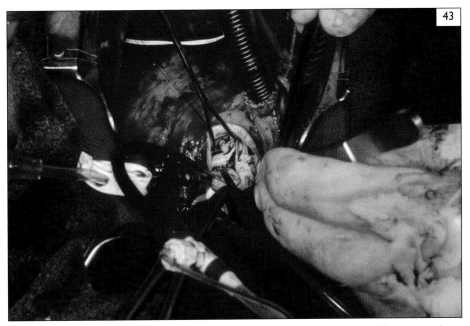

**43** Intraoperative photograph of a fibrocalcific, stenosed aortic valve. (Courtesy of John Sanders, MD.)

**Table 13** Recommendations for aortic valve replacement in aortic stenosis

| Indication | Class |
|---|---|
| Symptomatic patients with severe AS | I |
| Patients with severe AS undergoing coronary artery bypass surgery | I |
| Patients with severe AS undergoing surgery on the aorta or other heart valves | I |
| Patients with moderate AS undergoing coronary artery bypass surgery or surgery on the aorta or other heart valves (see sections III.F.6., III.F.7., and VIII.D. of these guidelines) | IIa |
| Asymptomatic patients with severe AS and LV systolic dysfunction | IIa |
| Abnormal response to exercise (e.g. hypotension) | IIa |
| Ventricular tachycardia | IIb |
| Marked or excessive LV hypertrophy(=15mm) | IIb |
| Valve area <0.6 cm$^2$ | IIb |
| Prevention of sudden death in asymptomatic patients with none of the findings listed under indication 5 | III |

AS: aortic stenosis; LV: left ventricular. (Adapted from Bonow RO, Carabello B, de Leon AC Jr, *et al.* (1998). ACC/AHA guidelines for the management of patients with valvular heart disease. *Journal of the American College of Cardiology* **32**:1486–1588.)

Though infrequently used, an operation which may be useful when AVR is not possible, is the creation of an apico-aortic conduit to the descending aorta. This procedure has been employed in the frail elderly deemed unlikely to survive AVR (Takemura, 2003; Crestanello *et al.*, 2004). The technique is illustrated in **44–51**.

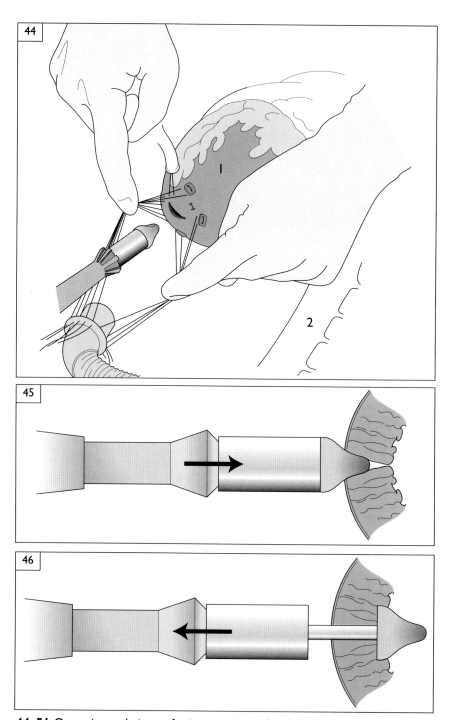

**44–51** Operative technique of apico-aortic conduit (very rarely employed today). 1: left ventricle; 2: descending aorta; 3: left atrium. (Courtesy of John W. Brown, MD.)

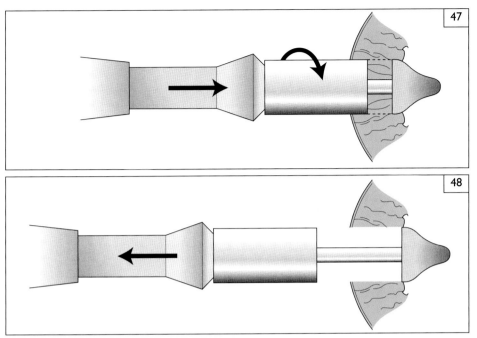

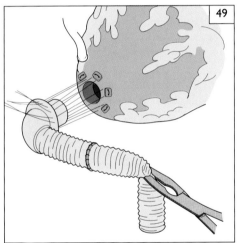

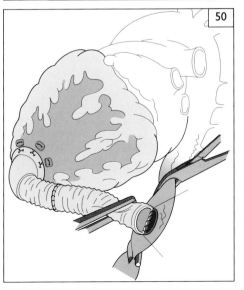

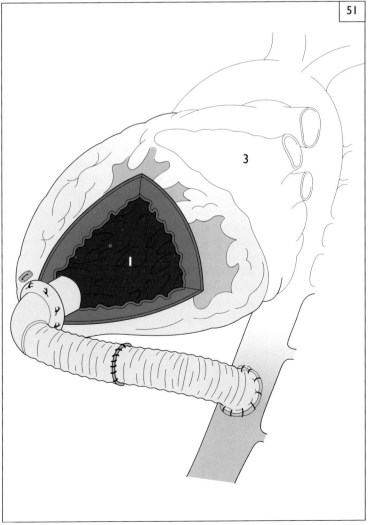

## Case study

A 55-year-old, single, male accountant scheduled an appointment with his family physician to discuss a new problem of shortness of breath. Over the previous 3–4 months, he noticed that he was 'losing his wind' during his noontime walk on a 2 mile loop near his office. Ten years earlier, when he first started working at this location, he had been able to cover this distance in 45 minutes. Because of increasing workload, he had stopped walking 5 years earlier, but had recently resumed this habit on the basis of a New Year's resolution. This loop now took him over 1 hour and he had to stop at the top of the modest hill on the route to catch his breath. On one or two occasions, when the weather was particularly cold, he had noticed some mild tightness in his chest. He had noticed infrequent swelling of his ankles that always resolved overnight. He denied any palpitations or syncope. He denied ever having rheumatic fever.

His past medical history was notable for a mild murmur heard during a military exam, but it did not prevent him from serving for 2 years in the Army. He also had mild hypertension and dyslipidemia, with his most recent lipid panel revealing triglycerides of 4.1 mmol/l (366 mg/dl), high-density cholesterol of 0.7 mmol/l (28 mg/dl), and low-density cholesterol of 3.8 mmol/l (145 mg/dl). His current medications included hydrocholorothiazide 25 mg daily, aspirin 81 mg daily.

With regard to his social history, he grew up in Illinois, but for the past 34 years he had worked in New England. He had always been single, had no children, smoked 1 pack per day throughout his 20s but none since, and drank 1–2 beers daily. There was no history of heart disease among his immediate family. He had three brothers and four sisters, all younger than he.

On exam, he was a balding, moderately obese man with a large mustache appearing comfortable while seated. His heart rate was 82 bpm and regular. His blood pressure was 165/95 mmHg (22/12.7 kPa) in both arms. Chest exam revealed good air movement without crackles or wheezes. His jugular venous pressure was estimated at 6 cm above the sternal angle, with a prominent a wave. A soft bruit was heard over the carotids, louder on the right side. The upstroke was diminished in amplitude and was slow to peak. His apical impulse, located in the 5th intercostal space in the midclavicular line, was approximately 5 cm in diameter and sustained. A subtle presystolic impulse was also palpable. A harsh, diamond-shaped, late-peaking systolic murmur was heard over the precordium. $S_1$ was normal; $S_2$ was

audible and snappy. An ejection sound was heard immediately following $S_1$. The Valsalva maneuver had no effect on the murmur. No diastolic murmur was heard during held end-expiration while leaning forward. His abdomen was unremarkable. He had palpable femoral pulses bilaterally. His feet were warm but pedal pulses were not palpable.

His ECG demonstrated sinus rhythm with left atrial and left ventricular hypertrophy, with asymmetrically inverted lateral T waves consistent with strain pattern. A complete blood count, electrolytes, renal function, thyroid reflex panel, and liver enzymes as well as a chest radiograph and echocardiogram were ordered.

One week later, the cardiologist reported the finding of severe AS, with a peak aortic velocity of 4.8 m/s, peak and mean gradients of 92 and 55 mmHg (12.3 and 7.3 kPa) respectively, a dimensionless obstructive index (ratio of LVOT velocity to Ao velocity) of 0.20, and an estimated aortic valve area of 0.8 cm². The aortic valve appeared to be bicuspid. The ventricle was moderately hypertrophied with a posterior wall and septal thickness of 15 mm. The LA was enlarged. Estimated pulmonary artery systolic pressure was 65 mmHg (8.7 kPa). From the suprasternal view, there was the suggestion of turbulent flow in the aorta just distal to the left subclavian take off.

After consultation with a cardiologist, the patient underwent left and right heart catheterization, coronary angiography, and ascending aortography. Elevated right- and left-sided pressures were confirmed, CO was normal at rest, and coronary angiography showed mild diffuse disease with an 80% focal narrowing in the distal dominant right coronary artery. Aortography revealed a mild coarctation of the aorta with a peak to peak pressure gradient of 20 mmHg (2.7 kPa). The valve was not crossed because the clinical and echocardiography data were congruent.

The patient underwent uncomplicated AVR with a mechanical bileaflet tilting prosthesis and a saphenous vein bypass from the aorta to the posterior descending artery. Six months later he was still walking at noon and had lost 11 kg (25 pounds). He was taking warfarin, but was closely following the development of direct thrombin inhibitors on the internet as a potential alternative not requiring monitoring.

COMMENTS

This case highlights some characteristics of a patient with a bicuspid aortic valve who develops severe stenosis. Of note, the ejection sound and snappy $S_2$ are very suggestive of a bicuspid valve. The other exam findings are representative of AS with LVH.

Coarctation is associated with bicuspid valves. It was not suspected because it was distal to the left subclavian, and lower extremity blood pressure was not checked. It was not repaired because it produced only modest hemodynamic effects. The echo data is all consistent with severe stenosis. The choice of a mechanical valve was influenced by the patient's dominant concern of avoiding reoperation.

## References

Braunwald E (2001). Valvular heart disease. In: *Heart Disease: A Textbook of Cardiovascular Medicine.* E Braunwald, DP Zipes, P Libby (eds). WB Saunders, Philadelphia, ch 46, pp. 1643–1722.

Carabello B (2002). Aortic stenosis. *New England Journal of Medicine* 346(9):677–682.

Chambers J, Bach D, Dumesnil J, Otto C, Shah P, Thomas J (2004). Crossing the aortic valve in severe aortic stenosis: no longer acceptable? *Journal of Heart Valve Disease* 13(3):344–346.

Crestanello JA, Zehr KJ, Daly RC, *et al.* (2004). Is there a role for the left ventricle apical-aortic conduit for acquired aortic stenosis? *Journal of Heart Valve Disease* 13(1):57–62.

Cribier A, Eltchaninoff H, Tron C (2003). [First human transcatheter implantation of an aortic valve prosthesis in a case of severe calcific aortic stenosis]. *Annales de Cardiologie et d'Angeiologie* 52(3):173–175.

Iung B, Gohlke-Bärwolf, Tornos P, *et al.* on behalf of the Working Group on Valvular Heart Disease (2002). Recommendations on the management of the asymptomatic patient with valvular heart disease. *European Heart Journal* 23(16):1253–1266.

Jamieson WRE, Edward FH, Schwartz M, *et al.* (1999). Risk stratification for cardiac valve replacement: national cardiac surgery database. *Annals of Thoracic Surgery* 67:943–951.

Juvonen J, Juvonen T, Laurila A, *et al.* (1998). Can degenerative aortic valve stenosis be related to persistent *Chlamydia pneumoniae* infection? *Annals of Internal Medicine* 128(9):741–744.

Kupfahl C, Honold M, Meinhardt G, *et al.* (2004). Evaluation of aortic stenosis by cardiovascular magnetic resonance imaging: comparison with established routine clinical techniques. *Heart* 90(8):893–901.

Leborgne L, Tribouilloy C, Otmani A, *et al.* (1998). Comparative value of Doppler echocardiography and cardiac catheterization in the decision to operate on patients with aortic stenosis. *International Journal of Cardiology* 65:163–168.

Lieberman EB, Bashore TM, Hermiller JB, *et al.* (1995). Balloon aortic valvularplasty in adults: failure of procedure to improve long-term survival. *Journal of the American College of Cardiology* 26:1522–1528.

Meine TJ, Harrison JK (2004). Should we cross the valve: the risk of retrograde catheterization of the left ventricle in patients with aortic stenosis. *American Heart Journal* 148(1):41–42.

Monin JL, Quere JP, Monchi M, *et al.* (2003). Low-gradient aortic stenosis: operative risk stratification and prediction of long-term outcome: a multi-center trial using dobutamine stress hemodynamics. *Circulation* 108(3):319–324.

Neithardt G, Sorrentino MJ (2003). *Etiology and natural history of mitral stenosis.* In: Up.To.Date.com BD Rose (ed). UpToDate, Wellesley, MA.

Nishimura RA (2000) Valvular stenosis In: *Mayo Clinic Cardiology Board Review.* JG Murphy (ed). Lippincott, Williams, and Wilkins, Philadelphia.

Novaro GM, Tioung IY, Pearce GL, *et al.* (2001). Effect of hydroxymethylglutaryl coenzyme A reductase inhibitors on the progression of calcific aortic stenosis. *Circulation* 104:2205–2209.

Okura H, Yoshida K, Hozumi T, *et al.* (1997). Planimetry and transthoracic two-dimensional echocardiography in noninvasive assessment of aortic valve area in patients with valvular aortic stenosis. *Journal of the American College of Cardiology* 30:753–759.

Otto CM (1999). Association of aortic valve stenosis with cardiovascular mortality and morbidity in the elderly. *New England Journal of Medicine* 341:142–147.

Otto CM, Kuusisto J, Reichenbach DD, *et al.* (1994). Characterization of the early lesion of 'degenerative' valvular aortic stenosis: histological and immunohistochemical studies. *Circulation* 90:844–853.

Peter M, Hoffmann A, Parker C, Luscher T, Burckhardt D (1993). Progression of aortic stenosis in adults: role of age and concomitant coronary disease. *Chest* 103:1715–1719.

Rosenhek R, Binder T, Porenta G, *et al.* (2000). Predictors of outcome in severe, asymptomatic aortic stenosis. *New England Journal of Medicine* 343(9):611–617.

Ross J, Braunwald E (1968). Aortic stenosis. *Circulation* 38(Suppl V):61–67.

Takemura T, Shimamura Y, Sakaguchi M, *et al.* (2003). [Apico-aortic conduit for severe aortic stenosis in the elderly.] *Japanese Journal of Thoracic Surgery* 56(13):1139–1143.

# Chapter Five

# Chronic Aortic Regurgitation

## Definition

Aortic regurgitation (AR) refers to blood flow from the aorta into the left ventricle (LV) during diastole. It is commonly classified as acute or chronic in light of their distinct clinical presentations. Chronic AR generally refers to valve lesions with a duration of months to years.

## Etiology

In contrast to aortic stenosis, the causes of AR are much more diverse. The primary defect may reside in the valve or in the aortic root. Primary valvular causes include unicuspid and bicuspid aortic valves, discrete subaortic stenosis (with high pressure jet-induced damage to the valve), ventricular septal defects with a prolapsing aortic cusp, rheumatic heart disease, calcific degeneration, myxomatous proliferation, Takayasu's disease, Whipple's disease, Crohn's disease, systemic lupus erythematous, infective endocarditis, aortic valve trauma, and connective tissue diseases including rheumatoid arthritis, giant cell aortitis, Reiter's syndrome, and ankylosing spondylitis.

Disorders associated with aortic root dilatation (52–54) include systemic hypertension, cystic medial degeneration of the aorta, senile aortic dilatation, annuloaortic ectasia, syphilis, osteogenesis imperfecta, Marfan syndrome, Ehler–Danlos syndrome, relapsing polychondritis, psoriatic arthritis, Behçet's syndrome, and ulcerative colitis-associated arthritis. Aortic dissection (55) results in aortic regurgitation by causing disruption of the cuspal attachments (Braunwald, 2001).

## Pathophysiology

In chronic AR, the LV is subject to a gradually increasing volume load. The gradual pace allows for a series of adaptations characterized by an increase in LV compliance and simultaneous chamber dilatation and wall thickening (eccentric hypertrophy). At a cellular level, this is accomplished by the addition of sarcomeres in series and the elongation of myocytes. Wall stress, a function of pressure and radius divided by wall thickness, is kept in check by increases in compliance, which reduces pressure at any given volume, and by wall thickening. LV dilatation serves to accommodate the increased regurgitant volume and maintains normal forward stroke volume despite a falling ejection fraction (EF). When the limits of increasing compliance and eccentric hypertrophy are reached, wall stress begins to rise. This represents an intolerable increase in afterload and leads to deteriorating systolic performance. This, in turn, leads to increasing end-diastolic volume and pressure accompanied by decreasing forward stroke volume, ultimately resulting in the syndrome of heart failure. In multiple studies, LV systolic function and end-systolic diameter have been identified as predictors of survival following aortic valve replacement (AVR) (Bonow et al., 1998).

## Clinical presentation

### SYMPTOMS

Initial symptoms are generally those of gradually developing fatigue, dyspnea on exertion, or angina. Rarely, sudden death is the first manifestation.

## Signs

There are many eponyms associated with physical findings in AR which originated in the preimaging era of cardiovascular medicine. The widened pulse pressure and increased stroke volume produce many distinctive features of the peripheral pulse. They include de Musset sign (head bobbing in rhythm with the pulse), Corrigan or water hammer pulse (abrupt upstroke and collapse of the palpated radial artery during elevation of the arm), Traube sign (systolic and diastolic pistol shot-like sounds heard over the femoral artery), Müller sign (systolic uvular movement), Duroziez sign (systolic bruit of the femoral artery upon proximal compression and diastolic bruit upon distal compression), and Quincke sign (capillary pulsations seen by transillumination of a finger tip or gentle compression of the lip with a glass slide).

Another sign of increased pulse pressure was recently described by ophthalmologists in the UK, whose recognition of increased ocular pulse amplitude led to the diagnosis of severe chronic AR. As expected, the ocular pulse amplitude returned to normal postoperatively (McKee *et al.*, 2004).

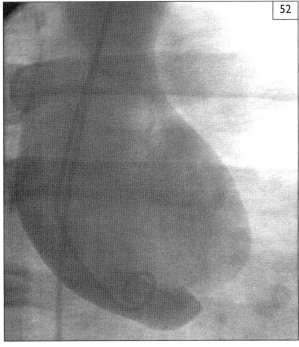

**52** Aortogram demonstrating massive dilatation of the aortic root and ascending aorta (annuloaortic ectasia).

**53, 54** Apical 4-chamber views of a patient with a dilated aortic root and associated severe aortic regurgitation. **53** 2D view highlighting the increased diameter of the aortic root and the left ventricle, resulting from the regurgitant volume.
**54** Color Doppler image of the regurgitant flow from aorta to left ventricle. 1: left ventricle; 2: right ventricle; 3: aortic root; 4: right atrium; 5: left atrium.

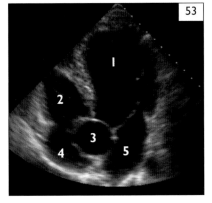

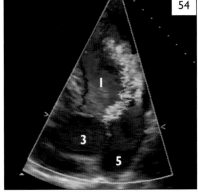

**55** Aortogram revealing the presence of an endothelial flap which narrows the true lumen through which the radiocontrast is flowing.

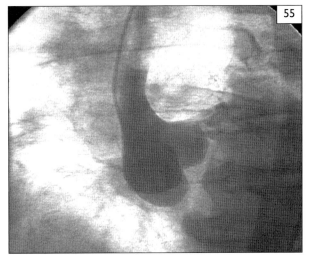

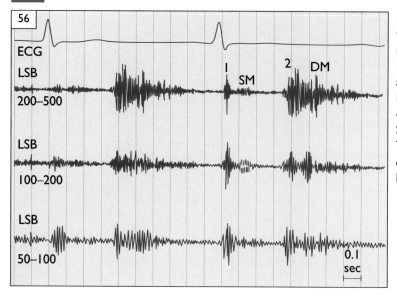

**56** Phonocardiogram demonstrating the characteristic decrescendo diastolic murmur of chronic aortic regurgitation. Note that the higher frequency sounds are of the greatest amplitude. DM: diastolic murmur; ECG: electrocardiogram; LSB: left sternal border; SM: systolic murmur. (Adapted from Tavel ME (1972). *Clinical Phonocardiography and External Pulse Recording.* Yearbook Medical Publishers, Chicago.)

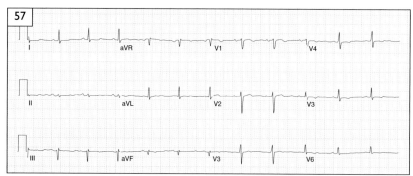

**57** 12-lead electrocardiogram from a patient with documented AR showing sinus rhythm and nonspecific ST-T abnormalities.

Palpation of the chest reveals an inferolaterally displaced, diffuse, hyperdynamic apical impulse often accompanied by a palpable, rapid filling wave at the apex and a systolic thrill at the base. Auscultation often discloses a systolic ejection sound and, with the development of LV failure, an $S_3$. The principal murmur is a high-pitched rapidly peaking diastolic murmur beginning immediately after $A_2$, heard best with the diaphragm while the patient leans forward in held end-expiration (**56**). Increasing regurgitant volume produces a progressively longer and coarser murmur. Eversion or perforation of an aortic cusp may produce a 'cooing dove' sound (Braunwald, 2001).

The location of the murmur provides some clue to the mechanism of the regurgitant flow. Valvular pathology usually produces a murmur along the left sternal border while aortic root dilatation generates a right sternal border murmur (Harvey *et al.*, 1963). Another murmur associated with chronic AR is the Austin Flint murmur, a mid-to-late diastolic rumble heard at the apex, arising from turbulent flow through a normal mitral valve being closed by the rapidly rising diastolic LV pressure. Finally, a short midsystolic ejection murmur may develop as a result of the increased stroke volume.

LABORATORY FINDINGS
The electrocardiogram (ECG) often shows evidence of LV hypertrophy (LVH) with strain which may include intraventricular conduction delay in advanced disease (**57**).

The chest X-ray typically demonstrates cardiomegaly in proportion to the duration and severity of AR. Ascending aortic dilatation is seen with associated aortic stenosis (AS) or connective tissue disease (**58, 59**).

Although rarely used as a primary diagnostic test, invasive hemodynamic evaluation by left heart catheterization (**60**) and aortic angiography (**61**) can be used to grade the severity of AR. Coronary angiography is generally used to identify concomitant coronary artery disease in patients in whom surgery is anticipated.

**58, 59** Postero-anterior and lateral chest films of a patient with severe aortic stenosis and aortic insufficiency. Note the increase in cardiothoracic ratio and the vascular prominence and peribronchial cuffing suggestive of pulmonary venous hypertension. (Courtesy of Bill Black, MD.)

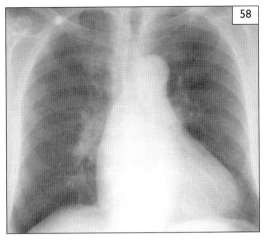

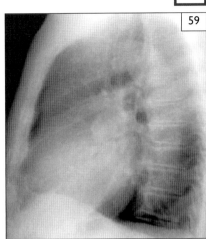

**60** Invasive hemodynamic tracing of aortic pressure (purple) from a patient with moderate (2+/4+) aortic regurgitation. Note the 94 mmHg (12.5 kPa) pulse pressure.

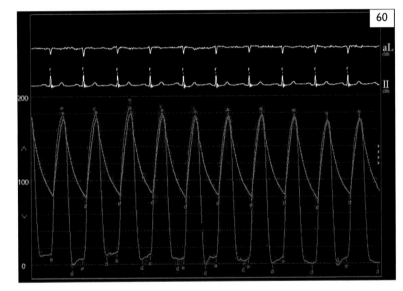

**61** Aortogram taken in right anterior oblique projection, demonstrating severe aortic regurgitation evidenced by the density of contrast which has regurgitated from the site of injection in the aortic root (note pigtail catheter) into the left ventricle.

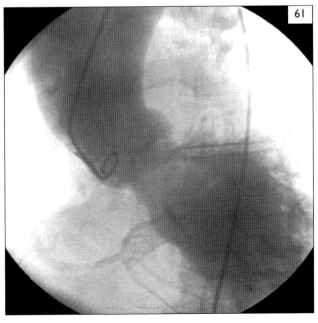

Echocardiography is the principal means of characterizing the mechanism, gauging the severity, and evaluating LV size and function in chronic AR. 2D imaging and Doppler interrogation both play important roles in the assessment (**62, 63**).

In the absence of any other regurgitant valves, radionuclide imaging can provide semiquantitative assessment of AR severity by comparison of right ventricular (RV) and LV stroke volumes. An LV to RV ratio of ≥2.0 indicates severe AR (Dehmer, 1981).

Finally, magnetic resonance imaging (MRI) is emerging as a reliable technique for evaluating AR (Kozerke *et al.*, 2001).

**Natural history**

The course of chronic regurgitation is typically indolent with a prolonged asymptomatic phase. During the asymptomatic phase, patients with severe AR and normal LV function develop symptoms, impaired LV function, or death at a rate of 3.7% per year. Relevant to follow-up, symptoms may not always precede LV dysfunction. Approximately 25% of patients with severe AR develop LV systolic dysfunction or die without antecedent symptoms.

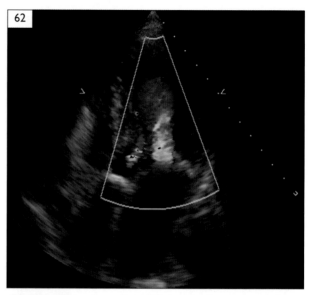

**62** Color Doppler echocardiography from an apical 4-chamber position showing regurgitant aortic flow (smaller orange flow) to the left and occuring simultaneously with antegrade mitral flow (larger orange flow seen on the right).

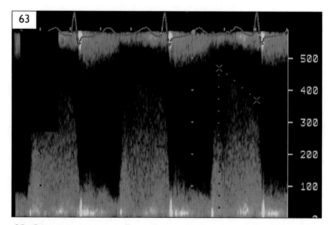

**63** Continuous wave Doppler interrogation of aortic regurgitant flow. Based on the rate of decline in velocity of this flow (indicated by the two X marks), estimates of the severity of regurgitation can be made.

In multivariate analyses, the only independent predictors of outcome based on initial evaluation are age and LV end-systolic dimension (Bonow *et al.*, 1998). The importance of intervening before LV dilatation develops is based on the observation that during a follow-up period of >8 years, patients with an end-systolic dimension of >50 mm had a 19% per year risk of symptoms, new LV dysfunction, or death; at 40–45 mm, the risk was 6% per year; and at <40 mm, the risk was zero (Bonow *et al.*, 1991). These observations highlight the importance of careful auscultation and serial imaging in the proper care of patients with chronic AR (discussed in more detail later in this chapter).

## Medical management
### MEDICAL THERAPY
In laboratory studies, the combination of hydralazine and sodium nitroprusside, as well as oral nifedipine have been shown to improve forward cardiac output and to decrease regurgitant volume. In clinical trials, only long-acting nifedipine, when compared to digoxin, has been proven to slow the progression of the disease (Scognamiglio *et al.*, 1994). This study examined patients with chronic, severe AR with LV dilatation but preserved systolic function. Currently, vasodilator therapy is indicated for this group, patients awaiting surgery, and patients who are not surgical candidates due to comorbidities (*Table 14*). The dose of nifedipine or hydralazine should be advanced until a drop in systolic pressure is noted. Normalization of systolic pressure is not the goal and attempts to do so may be hazardous. Patients who are normotensive at rest should not be treated with vasodilators (Bonow *et al.*, 1998).

### PHYSICAL ACTIVITY
There is no evidence that strenuous exercise is harmful in patients with asymptomatic AR and normal LV function. An exercise tolerance test is generally recommended prior to participating in athletics. Isometric exercise may be harmful. More detailed guidelines are available in the 26th Bethesda Conference (Cheitlin *et al.*, 1994).

**Table 14** Recommendations for vasodilator therapy for chronic aortic regurgitation

| Indication | Class |
| --- | --- |
| Chronic therapy in patients with severe regurgitation who have symptoms and/or LV dysfunction when surgery is not recommended because of additional cardiac or noncardiac factors | I |
| Long-term therapy in asymptomatic patients with severe regurgitation who have LV dilatation but normal systolic function | I |
| Long-term therapy in asymptomatic patients with hypertension and any degree of regurgitation | I |
| Long-term ACE inhibitor therapy patients with persistent LV systolic dysfunction after AVR | I |
| Short-term therapy to improve the hemodynamic profile of patients with severe heart failure symptoms and severe LV dysfunction before proceeding with AVR | I |
| Long-term therapy in asymptomatic patients with mild-to-moderate AR and normal LV systolic function | III |
| Long-term therapy in asymptomatic patients with LV systolic dysfunction who are otherwise candidates for valve replacement | III |
| Long-term therapy in symptomatic patients with either normal LV function or mild-to-moderate LV systolic dysfunction who are otherwise candidates for valve replacement | III |

ACE: angiotensin-converting enzyme; AR: aortic regurgitation; AVR: aortic valve replacement; LV: left ventricular. (Adapted from Bonow RO, Carabello B, de Leon AC Jr, *et al.* (1998). ACC/AHA guidelines for the management of patients with valvular heart disease. *Journal of the American College of Cardiology* **32**:1486–1588.)

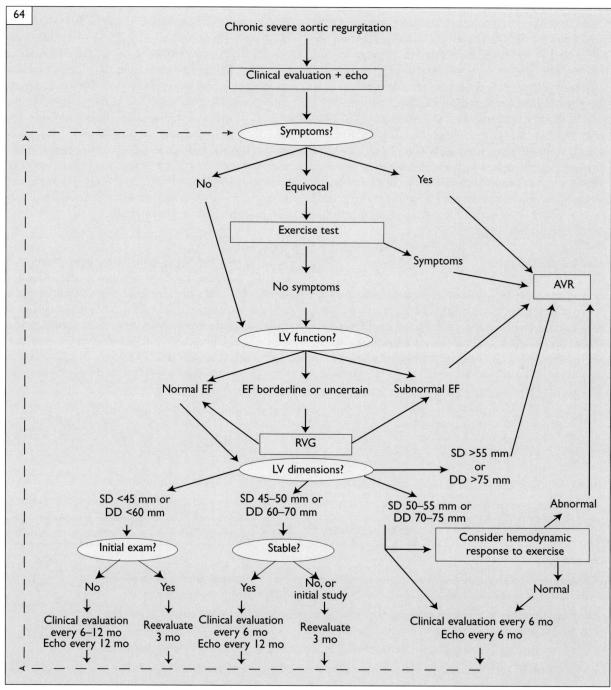

**64** Management strategy for patients with severe aortic regurgitation. Preoperative coronary angiography should be performed routinely as determined by age, symptoms, and coronary risk factors. Cardiac catheterization and angiography may also be helpful when there is discordance between clinical findings and echocardiography. In some centers, serial follow-up may be performed with radionuclide ventriculography (RVG) or magnetic resonance imaging (MRI) rather than echocardiography (echo) to assess LV volume and systolic function. AVR: aortic valve replacement; DD: end-diastolic dimension; EF: ejection fraction; LV: left ventricular; SD: end-systolic dimension. (Adapted from Bonow RO, Carabello B, de Leon AC Jr, *et al.* (1998). ACC/AHA guidelines for the management of patients with valvular heart disease. *Journal of the American College of Cardiology* **32**:1486–1588.)

## PATIENT FOLLOW-UP

All patients with AR require surveillance. This consists of periodic symptom review, physical examination, assessment of LV size and function, and selective use of exercise testing. Echocardiography is the most commonly used imaging technique but radionuclide ventriculograms (RVGs) or MRI may substitute in the event of poor echocardiographic images. The frequency of surveillance is dictated by the degree of LV dilatation and AR severity (**64**). The development of symptoms demands timely evaluation. Exercise testing may be helpful in patients with equivocal symptoms.

## Surgical intervention

### REPAIR VERSUS REPLACEMENT

Although repair of mitral valves due to myxomatous disease is well established as a safe and effective treatment, the traditional approach to regurgitation in the aortic position has been valve replacement. To date, attempts to repair aortic valves have met with limited success. In a recently reported series of 21 children undergoing valve repair between 1990 and 2000 with a mean follow up of 5.3 years, 47% clearly failed and required reoperation and valve replacement (Hasaniya *et al.*, 2004). Another recently described series reported the midterm results of valve repair (primarily aortic cusp extension with glutaraldehyde-treated autologous pericardial tissue) in patients with rheumatic AR. In this series, 9 of 46 patients (19.6%) followed for a mean of 4.6 years needed reoperation with valve replacement (Bozbuga *et al.*, 2004). Another recent single center series focused on repair of bicuspid aortic valves. In a retrospective, matched cohort analysis of 44 patients undergoing repair and followed for 2.6 yrs, the freedom from moderate or severe AR was 79% in the repair group vs. 94% in the valve replacement group, with no thromboembolic events in either group (Davierwala *et al.*, 2003). Finally, the results of 11 surgical series involving a total of 761 patients who underwent repair between 1990 and 2002 were recently summarized. The reoperation rates for repair were 89% and 64% at 5 and 10 years respectively (Carr and Savage, 2004).

### ASYMPTOMATIC PATIENTS

Although some debate persists, most US experts recommend AVR for asymptomatic patients who develop: (i) LV systolic dysfunction as documented by two separate imaging studies; and (ii) patients with severe LV dilatation (end-systolic diameter >55 mm or end-diastolic diameter >75 mm). The European Society of Cardiology (ESC) guidelines recommend slightly more aggressive surgical criteria: absolute end-systolic and end-diastolic diameters of 50 and 70 mm, respectively. The ESC also emphasizes the value of indexing to body surface area and proposes consideration of surgical intervention at an end-systolic dimension of >25 mm/m$^2$. It is recognized that this criterion will be reached before the nonindexed end-systolic dimension of 55 mm, but the recommendation is justified by the good outcomes seen especially in younger, thinner patients. Operative mortality in asymptomatic patients is low (1–3%) with long-term survival comparable to the general population with excellent functional results (Iung *et al.*, 2002). Some investigators have noted that women appear to do less well than men (Klodas *et al.*, 1996) which European experts cite as evidence supporting the value of indexing end-systolic dimension. Because of their smaller size, applying an absolute dimension threshold to women will result in surgery at a more advanced degree of LV dilatation than when measured by body surface area (BSA) indexed measures.

Surgical indications for aortic root replacement (65) have been outlined in the European guidelines since ascending aortic and aortic root dilatation often accompany AR (66). These indications include an aortic root diameter exceeding 55 mm (regardless of degree of AR), exceeding 50 mm in patients with bicuspid valves or Marfan' syndrome, or an ascending aortic diameter exceeding 55 mm in non-Marfan patients undergoing surgery for severe AR. Consistent with the reasoning above, European guidelines also recommend consideration of body surface area and suggest ascending aortic replacement when the observed to predicted aortic root diameter ratio exceeds 1.3. For patients older than 40 years, aortic root diameter is predicted as $1.92 + (0.74 \times BSA)$ (Roman *et al.*, 1993).

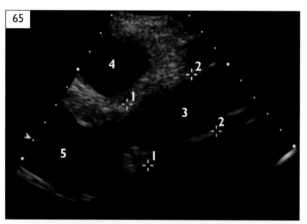

**65** Parasternal long axis view of a patient who had undergone combined aortic valve and ascending aortic reconstruction with a valved conduit (Bental procedure). Note the increased wall thickness of the graft (lying between points 1 and 2) compared to the native ascending aorta (3) above. 4: right ventricle; 5: left ventricle.

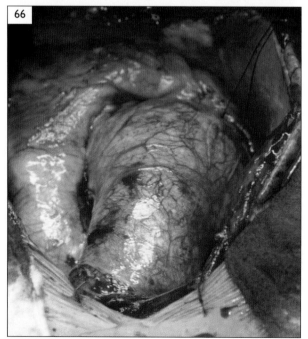

**66** Intraoperative view from the perspective of the anesthesiologist of a patient with severe annuloaortic ectasia with associated severe aortic regurgitation. (Courtesy of John Sanders, MD.)

## Symptomatic patients with normal left ventricular function

Symptoms which suggest the need for AVR include heart failure greater than New York Heart Association class II or angina severity greater than Canadian Cardiovascular Society class I. Clinical judgement is obviously required in the assessment of patients approaching, but not yet meeting, these surgical criteria. Orthopnea due to AR is always an indication for surgery.

## Symptomatic patients with left ventricular dysfunction

The decision to refer for surgery is straightforward in symptomatic patients with EF between 25 and 50%. In patients with an EF <25% or an end-systolic dimension >60 mm, the decision is more difficult because of the possibility of irreversible myocardial damage and high operative mortality. However, in most cases, valve replacement provides a better prognosis than medical therapy. Clearly, patients' preferences, expectations, and comorbidities factor heavily into the decision making (**64**, *Table 15*).

---

**Table 15** Recommendations for aortic valve replacement in chronic severe aortic regurgitation

| Indication | Class |
|---|---|
| Patients with NYHA functional Class III or IV symptoms and preserved LV systolic function, defined as normal EF at rest (EF =0.50) | I |
| Patients with NYHA functional Class II symptoms and preserved LV systolic function (EF =0.50 at rest) but with progressive LV dilatation or declining EF at rest on serial studies or declining effort tolerance on exercise testing | I |
| Patients with Canadian Heart Association functional Class II or greater angina with or without CAD | I |
| Asymptomatic or symptomatic patients with mild to moderate LV dysfunction at rest (EF 0.25–0.49) | I |
| Patients undergoing coronary artery bypass surgery or surgery on the aorta or other heart valves | I |
| Patients with NYHA functional Class II symptoms and preserved LV systolic function (EF =0.50 at rest) with stable LV size and systolic function on serial studies and stable exercise tolerance | IIa |
| Asymptomatic patients with normal LV systolic function (EF >0.50) but with severe LV dilatation (end-diastolic dimension >75 mm or end-systolic dimension >55 mm)* | IIa |
| Patients with severe LV dysfunction (EF <0.25) | IIb |
| Asymptomatic patients with normal systolic function at rest (EF >0.50) and progressive LV dilatation when the degree of dilatation is moderately severe (end-diastolic dimension 70–75 mm, end-systolic dimension 50–55 mm) | IIb |
| Asymptomatic patients with normal systolic function at rest (EF >0.50) but with decline in EF during: | |
|     Exercise radionuclide angiography | IIb |
|     Stress echocardiography | III |
| Asymptomatic patients with normal systolic function at rest (EF >0.50) and LV dilatation when degree of dilatation is not severe (end-diastolic dimension <70 mm, end-systolic dimension <50 mm) | III |

*Consider lower threshold values for patients of small stature of either gender. Clinical judgement is required.
CAD: coronary artery disease; EF: ejection fraction; LV: left ventricular; NYHA: New York Heart Association.
(Adapted from Bonow RO, Carabello B, de Leon AC Jr, *et al.* (1998). ACC/AHA guidelines for the management of patients with valvular heart disease. *Journal of the American College of Cardiology* **32**:1486–1588.)

## Case study

A 46-year-old female former college volleyball player sought medical attention from her physician because of gradually increasing fatigue. After having enjoyed a terrific exercise tolerance for all of young adulthood, she had noticed the slow development of shortness of breath during activity. Six months earlier she had become very winded while rowing on the local river. She attributed this to the unfamiliar type of exercise. However, she now noticed that she became winded when carrying groceries up the stairs from her garage, and would sometimes develop a dry cough. In addition, her heart seemed to pound more forcefully in her chest with normal activities. She denied any chest discomfort, syncope, orthopnea, ankle edema, fever, or chills.

Her past medical history was notable for two uneventful pregnancies and an uncomplicated appendectomy at age 17 years. She took no medications. She was married with two children and worked in an advertising office. Her parents were well. She had no siblings.

On exam, she was 2 m (6' 6") tall and weighed 69 kg (154 lb). Her lower body appeared longer than her upper body; she had narrow wrists and long, mildly tapered fingers. Her head subtly bobbed in concert with her pulse. Her blood pressure was 160/55 mmHg (21.3/7.3 kPa) in both arms and her pulse was 70 bpm and regular. Her pulse was of high amplitude with a rapid run off. Transillumination of her fingertips revealed capillary pulsations. Her skin was warm and dry. Her uvula also moved in tempo with her pulse. Her chest was clear to percussion and auscultation and demonstrated a mild pectus excavatum. Estimated right atrial pressure was 6 cm of $H_2O$ with normal venous pulsations. There were no carotid bruits. Her apical impulse was hyperdynamic and displaced to the 6th intercostal space in the anterior axillary line. An $S_3$ was palpable over the apex and a thrill was appreciated at the right upper sternal border. On auscultation, there was an $S_3$ at the apex, a grade 3/6 midsystolic murmur loudest at the base, and a grade 2/6 early diastolic murmur radiating along the right sternal border. The remainder of the exam was unremarkable.

An ECG performed during the visit documented sinus rhythm with voltage criteria for LVH and a mild intraventricular conduction delay. Her chest film revealed a widened upper mediastinum and a cardiac to lateral thoracic diameter ratio of >0.5. Blood counts, electrolytes, renal function, and sedimentation rates were all within normal limits.

An echocardiogram revealed annuloaortic ectasia with severe AR. The pressure half-time of aortic flow deceleration was 210 msec and holodiastolic flow reversal was seen in the abdominal aorta. The LV was dilated with an end-diastolic internal diameter of 7.7 cm. Systolic function was mildly impaired, with a visually estimated ejection fraction of 45%. Long-acting nifedipine was initiated at a dose of 30 mg/day and cardiology consultation was requested.

After a right and left heart catheterization with coronary and ascending aortic angiography confirming severe AR and normal coronary anatomy, the patient underwent replacement of the aortic valve and ascending aorta. The surgeon employed an integrated mechanical valve and tube graft with reimplantation of the patient's coronaries to the tube graft. The patient's hospital course was complicated by postoperative atrial fibrillation and a transient ischemic attack. Two months after surgery, she was feeling well and her LV end-diastolic diameter was decreased to 6.5 cm.

## COMMENTS

This case highlights the association of Marfan's syndrome with dilatation of the ascending aorta which, in turn, is often complicated by aortic insufficiency. This patient had reached the usual threshold for surgical intervention; the nifedipine was used in the hope of slowing progression while surgical planning was undertaken. Because the patient had a systemic defect in connective tissue, a decision was made to completely excise and replace the aortic valve, sinus, and ascending aorta. Her complications remind readers that an uneventful course cannot be assumed.

## References

Bonow RO, Lakatos E, Maron BJ, Epstein SE (1991). Serial long-term assessment of the natural history of asymptomatic patients with chronic aortic regurgitation and normal left ventricular systolic function. *Circulation* 84:1625–1635.

Bonow RO, Carabello B, de Leon AC Jr, *et al.* (1998). ACC/AHA guidelines for the management of patients with valvular heart disease: a report of the American College of Cardiology/American Heart Association Task Force on Practice Guidelines (Committee on Management of Patients with Valvular Heart Disease). *Journal of the American College of Cardiology* 32:1486–1588.

Bozbuga N, Erentug V, Kirali K, Akinci E, Isik O, Yakut C (2004). Midterm results of aortic valve repair with the pericardial cusp extension technique in rheumatic valve disease. *Annals of Thoracic Surgery* 77(4):1272–1276.

Braunwald E (2001). Valvular heart disease. In: *Heart Disease: A Textbook of Cardiovascular Medicine.* E Braunwald, DP Zipes, P Libby (eds). WB Saunders, Philadelphia, ch 46, pp. 1643–1722.

Carr JA, Savage EB (2004). Aortic valve repair for aortic insufficiency in adults: a contemporary review and comparison with replacement techniques. *European Journal of Cardiothoracic Surgery* 25(1):6–15.

Cheitlin MD, Douglas PS, Parmley WW (1994). 26th Bethesda conference: recommendations for determining eligibility for competition in athletes with cardiovascular abnormalities. Task Force 2: acquired valvular heart disease. *Journal of the American College of Cardiology* 24:874–880.

Davierwala PM, David TE, Armstrong S, Ivanov J (2003). Aortic valve repair versus replacement in bicuspid aortic valve disease. *Journal of Heart Valve Disease* 12(6):679–686; discussion 686.

Dehmer GH, Firth EG, Hillis LD, *et al.* (1981). Alterations in left ventricular volumes and ejection fraction at rest and during exercise in patients with aortic regurgitation. *American Journal of Cardiology* 48:17–27.

Harvey WP, Corrado MA, Perloff JK (1963). Right sided murmurs of aortic insufficiency (diastolic murmurs better heard to the right of the sternum rather than the left). *American Journal of Medical Science* 61:533–542.

Hasaniya N, Gundry SR, Razzouk AJ, Mulla N, Bailey LL (2004). Outcome of aortic valve repair in children with congenital aortic valve insufficiency. *Journal of Thoracic and Cardiovascular Surgery* 127(4):970–974.

Iung B, Gohlke-Bärwolf C, Tornos P, *et al.* on behalf of the Working Group on Valvular Heart Disease (2002). Recommendations on the management of the asymptomatic patient with valvular heart disease. *European Heart Journal* 23(16):1253–1266.

Klodas E, Enriquez-Sarano M, Tajik AJ, Mullany CJ, Bailey KR, Seward JB (1996). Surgery for aortic regurgitation in women. Contrasting indications and outcomes compared with men. *Circulation* 94:2472–2478.

Kozerke S, Scwitter J, Pederson EM, Boesiger P (2001). Aortic and mitral regurgitation: quantification using moving slice velocity mapping. *Journal of Magnetic Resonance Imaging* 14(2):106–112.

McKee HD, Saldana M, Ahad MA (2004). Increased ocular pulse amplitude revealing aortic regurgitation. *American Journal of Ophthalmology* 138(3):503.

Roman RJ, Rosen SE, Kramer-Fox R, *et al.* (1993). Prognostic significance of the pattern of aortic root dilation in the Marfan syndrome. *Journal of the American College of Cardiology* 22:1470–1476.

Scognamiglio R, Rahimtoola SH, Fasoli G, Nistri S, Dalla Volta S (1994). Nifedipine in asymptomatic patients with severe aortic regurgitation and normal left ventricular function. *New England Journal of Medicine* 331:689–694.

# Chapter Six

# Acute Aortic Regurgitation

### Definition

Aortic regurgitation (AR) refers to blood flow from the aorta into the left ventricle (LV) during diastole, caused by the incompetence of the aortic valve. Acute AR generally refers to pathology present for hours to days.

### Etiology

Acute AR can be caused by infective endocarditis, aortic dissection (67–71), acute hypertension, trauma, failure of prosthetic valves (Morocutti *et al.*, 2002) and, in rare cases, failure of congenitally abnormal valve cusps. In infective endocarditis, valvular insufficiency can result from a number of possible mechanisms, including perforation of the aortic cusps, disruption of the valve leaflets by bulky vegetations, and the formation of perivalvular fistulae.

In aortic dissection, the presence of aortic insufficiency implies that the dissection has extended to the level of the root (where the cusps attach at the sinotubular ridge) or to the level of the valvular annulus. In severe, acute hypertension, extraordinary increases in afterload overwhelm the integrity of the valve cusp and allow regurgitant flow that often reverses upon control of the hypertension, unless permanent damage has been done to the valve structures. In trauma, insufficiency can result from both tears of the cusps and avulsions of the annulus, which appear to occur at approximately equal frequencies (Unal *et al.*, 2001). These injuries are believed to result from the sudden increase in intrathoracic pressure during diastole, whereby blood is forced across the closed aortic valve. Blunt trauma occurring in deceleration injuries is the most common, but it has been described in the context of severe muscular exertion (childbirth and exercise) and following the kick of a horse (Leonard *et al.*, 1955). Spontaneous rupture of a valve cusp is rare, but it appears to occur in congenitally abnormal valves, especially those subjected to chronic hypertension (Blaszyk *et al.*, 1999). As of 1999, there were eight reported cases of spontaneous rupture of a fenestrated aortic cusp.

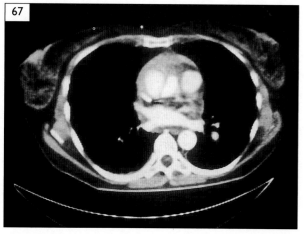

**67** Computed tomographic image through the upper mediastinum of a patient with dissection of the ascending aorta, a condition commonly associated with acute aortic regurgitation. Note the separate lumens in the ascending aorta.

## Pathophysiology

In acute AR, the LV is subject to a sudden increase in volume with no opportunity for the compensatory increase in compliance and the eccentric hypertrophy seen in chronic regurgitation. Without these adaptations of dilatation and increased compliance, pressure within the LV rapidly equilibrates with that of the aorta. The sharp increase in LV end-diastolic pressure leads to premature closure of the mitral valve. However, this is insufficient to protect the pulmonary venous circulation from the elevated pressure. This venous hypertension typically causes vascular congestion, interstitial edema and, if severe, alveolar flooding.

The severity of acute AR will depend upon the volume of regurgitation and the preexisting compliance of the ventricle. The volume of regurgitation, in turn, is influenced by three factors: the size of the regurgitant orifice, the duration of diastole, and the diastolic pressure gradient across the aortic valve. With this in mind, it is apparent that tachycardia, by limiting diastole, is a physiologic compensation to AR and should not be treated. In addition, hypertension would be expected to aggravate AR and should be treated.

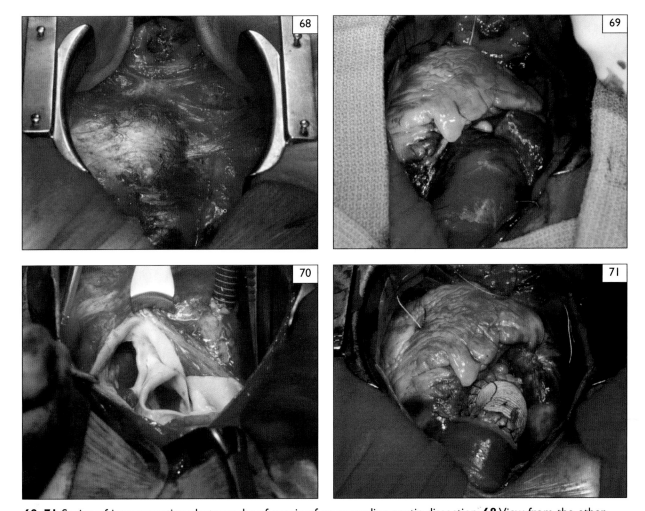

**68–71** Series of intraoperative photographs of repair of an ascending aortic dissection. **68** View from the ether screen with the pericardium intact. **69** Pericardium reflected revealing view of the ascending aorta. **70** Aorta transected revealing the true and false lumens. **71** Final result of graft placement in the ascending aorta. (Courtesy of John Sanders, MD.)

## Clinical presentation

### SYMPTOMS

The symptoms of acute AR will vary with both the underlying cause and the degree of valvular insufficiency. In cases of mild AR, there may be no symptoms of heart failure and the presentation will be dominated by the initiating event (e.g. endocarditis, aortic dissection, trauma). However, in the case of severe AR, the symptoms of heart failure will be prominent. They include the sudden onset of severe dypsnea, orthopnea, diaphoresis, and a sense of doom.

### SIGNS

Because the LV has not had time to remodel, the physical findings are distinct from those of chronic AR. If severe, the patient may be in extremis with a normal pulse pressure. Examination of the peripheral pulse may reveal the subtle finding of a rapidly rising pressure wave. The precordial impulse is typically hyperdynamic and only slightly displaced to the left. $S_1$ is usually soft due to premature closure of the mitral valve, $P_2$ will be loud in the presence of pulmonary hypertension, and an $S_3$ is common. Rapid equilibration between the LV and aorta results in a short diastolic murmur heard best with the patient leaning forward and holding his breath in end-expiration. An Austin Flint murmur, arising from the preclosure of the mitral valve, may be heard in mid-diastole over the mitral area. Chest examination often reveals tachypnea, diffuse inspiratory crackles and, if severe, frothy pink sputum.

Evaluation of a trauma patient with multiple injuries is particularly challenging. A high index of suspicion must be maintained, since the symptoms and findings may be subtle, and the examiner may be distracted by more obvious injuries (Munshi et al., 1996).

### LABORATORY FINDINGS

Chest X-ray findings include vascular congestion and alveolar edema with a normal sized heart. Electrocardiography generally reveals tachycardia and may display nonspecific or frankly ischemic appearing ST-T abnormalities. Echocardiography is the most valuable tool, providing color flow Doppler evidence of regurgitant flow through the aortic valve and Doppler evidence of rapid equilibration. Diastolic flutter of the anterior leaflet of the mitral valve is a classic M-mode echocardiographic feature and likely corresponds to the Austin Flint murmur. Preclosure of the mitral valve is another common finding. Transthoracic echocardiography may provide sufficient resolution to identify the mechanism of regurgitant flow. Most often transesophageal echocardiography (TEE) is necessary to characterize the valve pathology fully and is especially useful in critically ill patients.

If it does not delay urgent surgery, coronary catheterization and angiography should be performed (Rahimtoola, 1993). An invasive evaluation may serve to confirm the diagnosis in ambiguous cases, and may identify coexisting coronary artery disease which may be addressed at the time of valve surgery. This is particularly true in aortic dissection where the dissection may extend proximally to compromise a coronary ostium.

The hemodynamic findings of acute AR are distinct from those of chronic AR. Based on a comparison of nine patients with acute AR undergoing aortic valve replacement to a larger group of patients with chronic AR, the following observations were made: pulse pressure was much smaller ($55\pm7$ mmHg [$7.3\pm0.9$ kPa] vs. $105\pm22$ mmHg [$14\pm2.9$ kPa]), left ventricular end-diastolic volume (LVEDV) was smaller ($146\pm28$ vs. $264\pm64$ ml/m$^2$), stroke volume was smaller ($89\pm22$ vs. $163\pm57$ ml/m$^2$). In addition, the degree of mitral valve premature closure reflected the increase in left ventricular end-diastolic pressure (LVEDP) (Mann et al., 1975).

## Natural history

The natural history of acute AR will also vary with the severity and the underlying etiology. Stable small or moderate sized regurgitant orifices may be well tolerated. With medical therapy, the adaptations of chronic AR may allow the patient to defer or possibly avoid surgery altogether. However, in acute AR of a severe degree, patients will usually die of progressive heart failure in hours to days.

## Medical management

In severe heart failure, pharmacologic therapy serves only to support the patient until the surgical team is assembled. Diuretics, vasodilator therapy (e.g. nitroprusside) and positive inotropes (e.g. dopamine or dobutamine) may help to limit pulmonary venous hypertension and maintain cardiac output in the short term. Though commonly used in aortic dissection, beta-blockers may lead to circulatory collapse by inhibiting the compensatory tachycardia and should therefore be avoided (Bonow et al., 1998).

In AR associated with mild heart failure, these drugs may allow the patient to reach a compensated state of chronic AR. However, they will require ongoing surveillance for the development of pathologic LV dilatation or systolic dysfunction (see Chapter 5).

## Surgical intervention

Acute severe aortic regurgitation usually requires urgent valve replacement. In cases of aortic dissection, repair of the ascending aorta or replacement with a valved conduit may be necessary. The choice of valve prosthesis depends largely on the patient's life expectancy and any preexisting indication for anticoagulation. Older age and the absence of a separate need for anticoagulation (e.g. atrial fibrillation, recurrent deep vein thrombosis, preexisting mechanical valve) favor the use of a bioprosthesis. Conversely, younger age and separate need for anticoagulation favor the use of a mechanical valve prosthesis.

## Case study

A 60-year-old male truck mechanic was in his usual state of health until the day of admission; then while pulling hard on a rusted bolt, he developed the sudden onset of severe substernal chest discomfort. He couldn't describe the pain beyond saying 'it hurt awful bad'. The pain began at its full intensity. Over the course of the next hour, he became increasingly sweaty and short of breath. His fellow employees eventually convinced him to be transported to the emergency room.

His past medical history was notable for long-standing, poorly controlled hypertension, type 2 diabetes mellitus, obesity, and a 2 pack per day cigarette smoking habit. He also drank 6–12 beers per evening.

In the Emergency Department, he was anxious looking with a heart rate of 135 bpm and a blood pressure of 188/110 mmHg (25.1/14.7 kPa). He was diaphoretic with cool hands and feet. His right atrial pressure was estimated at 15 cm of $H_2O$. Inspiratory crackles were heard to the apices of both lungs and he had a wet cough. His point of maximal intensity (PMI) was not displaced, but was hyperdynamic with a palpable $S_3$. $S_1$ was soft and $P_2$ was loud. A short early diastolic murmur was heard along the left sternal border, and a middiastolic murmur was audible in the mitral area.

Chest X-ray revealed bilateral, perihilar, alveolar opacification with apical vascular engorgement and Kerley B lines. There was no cardiomegaly. ECG was remarkable for a sinus tachycardia and inferior ST segment elevation. An emergent echocardiogram demonstrated severe AR, characterized by a broad regurgitant flow jet relative to the left ventricular outflow tract diameter and a shortened pressure half-time of declining aortic antegrade flow. The inferior wall was akinetic. The patient was intubated and a transesophageal echocardiogram was performed, confirming the severe AR and identifying a dissection flap starting in the aortic root and extending into the descending thoracic aorta.

The patient was taken immediately to surgery, where the dissection was seen to extend into the root, disrupting the attachment of the right and noncoronary cusps and compressing the ostia of the right coronary artery. The patient was put on femoral artery cardiopulmonary bypass, and underwent replacement of the aortic valve and ascending aorta, with a valved conduit and reimplantation of the right coronary artery.

His postoperative course was complicated by delirium and a urinary tract infection. However, 4 months later he was back at work. He had stopped drinking, his blood pressure was well controlled, and his last echo showed an ejection fraction of 55% with mild inferior wall hypokinesis.

COMMENTS

This gentleman presumably had alcohol related hypertension complicated by an ascending aortic dissection. The dissection precipitated severe AR and an acute ST elevation myocardial infarction. The patient fortunately made it to a hospital with adequate resources to handle promptly this catastrophe. Symptoms and laboratory and imaging findings commonly seen in acute severe AR are noted.

## References

Blaszyk H, Witkiewicz AK, Edwards WD (1999). Acute aortic regurgitation due to spontaneous rupture of a fenestrated cusp. *Cardiovascular Pathology* 8(4):213–216.

Bonow RO, Carabello B, de Leon AC Jr, *et al.* (1998). ACC/AHA guidelines for the management of patients with valvular heart disease: a report of the American College of Cardiology/American Heart Association Task Force on Practice Guidelines (Committee on Management of Patients with Valvular Heart Disease). *Journal of the American College of Cardiology* 32:1486–1588.

Leonard JJ, Harvey WD, Hufnagel CA (1955). Rupture of the aortic valve: a therapeutic approach. *New England Journal of Medicine* 252:208–212.

Mann T, McLaurin L, Grossman W, *et al.* (1975). Assessing the hemodynamic severity of acute aortic regurgitation due to infective endocarditis. *New England Journal of Medicine* 293(3):108–113.

Morocutti G, Bernardi G, Gelsomino S (2002). Prosthetic valve dysfunction presenting as intermittent acute aortic regurgitation. *Heart* 88(1):3.

Munshi IA, Barie PS, Hawes AS, *et al.* (1996). Diagnosis and management of acute aortic valvular disruption secondary to rapid-deceleration trauma. *Journal of Trauma* 41(6):1047–1050.

Rahimtoola SH (1993). Recognition and management of acute aortic regurgitation. *Heart Disease and Stroke* 2:217–221.

Unal M, Demirsoy E, Gogus A, Arbatli H, Hamzaoglu A, Sonmez B (2001). Acute aortic valve regurgitation secondary to blunt chest trauma. *Texas Heart Institute Journal* 28(4):312–314.

# Chapter Seven

# Mitral Stenosis

## Definition

Mitral stenosis (MS) refers to flow limiting constriction of the mitral valve. The orifice of a normal mitral valve is 4.0–5.0 cm$^2$. Symptoms generally do not develop until the orifice is restricted to <2.5 cm$^2$. Valve areas of 1.5–2.5 cm$^2$ with mean pressure gradients <5 mmHg (0.7 kPa) are considered mild. Valve areas of 1.0–1.5 cm$^2$ or mean pressure gradients 5–10 mmHg (0.7–1.3 kPa) are considered moderate. Valve areas of <1.0 cm$^2$ or mean gradients >10 mmHg (1.3 kPa) are considered severe.

## Etiology

The majority of MS cases are related to rheumatic fever and disproportionately affect women (72, 73). Much less common causes include congenital valve malformations, carcinoid tumors, systemic lupus erythematosus, rheumatoid arthritis, Hunter–Hurler mucopolysaccharoidoses, Fabry disease, Whipple disease, and methysergide therapy.

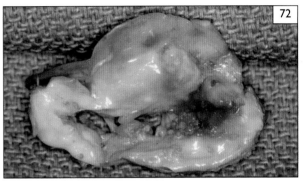

**72** An excised mitral valve from a patient with mitral stenosis due to rheumatic heart disease. The patient presented with transient ischemic attacks. (Courtesy of John Sanders, MD.)

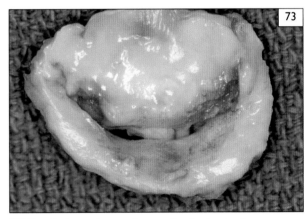

**73** Surgical specimen of an excised mitral valve from a patient with rheumatic heart disease and mitral stenosis. (Courtesy of John Sanders, MD.)

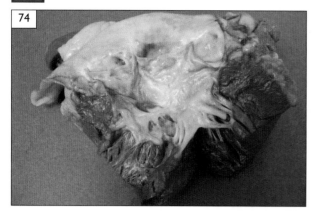

**74** The mitral valve is difficult to discern in this patient with rheumatic heart disease. The anterior and posterior leaflets lie below the aortic valve and are contracted and distorted. Note the accompanying mild fibrosis and coalescence of the subvalvular apparatus. (Courtesy of Nora Ratcliff, MD.)

## Pathophysiology

In rheumatic MS, exudative and proliferative inflammation of the underlying connective tissue leads to leaflet thickening and calcification, as well as commissural and chordal fusion (74–76). Ultimately, many patients are left with a funnel-shaped mitral apparatus (Roberts and Perloff, 1972).

As the mitral orifice narrows, left atrial (LA) pressure rises in response to less complete emptying and more vigorous atrial contraction (77). This elevated pressure increases the transmitral flow. However, the consequence of the elevated LA pressure is elevated pulmonary venous pressure which, in turn, produces pulmonary edema when hydrostatic forces exceed serum oncotic forces. With chronic exposure, the pulmonary arteriolar circulation responds with vasoconstriction, intimal hyperplasia, and medial hypertrophy, the histologic substrate of fixed pulmonary hypertension.

Since systole occupies a relatively fixed interval, it is predominantly diastole which shortens with rising heart rates. Clinically, this translates into less time available for transmitral flow and rising pressure gradients. By this mechanism, pulmonary vascular congestion and dyspnea often accompany an increase in heart rate in patients with MS.

## Clinical presentation

### SYMPTOMS

The most common presenting symptom is exertional dyspnea, often with accompanying cough, wheezing, orthopnea, and paroxysmal nocturnal dyspnea. Hemoptysis is common in severe disease. Other common presentations include chest pain, atrial

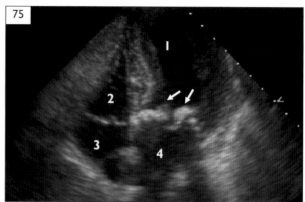

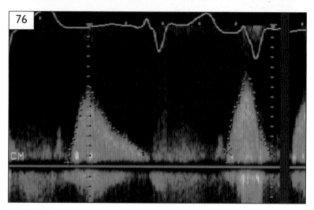

**75, 76** Severe calcific mitral stenosis. **75** Apical 4-chamber 2D image demonstrating severely calcified and thickened mitral leaflets (arrows). Note the black acoustic 'shadows' cast by the impenetrable calcified leaflets. 1: left ventricle; 2: right ventricle; 3: right atrium; 4: left atrium. **76** Continuous wave Doppler interrogation of antegrade flow across the valve reveals functional obstruction to flow with an estimated mean gradient of 6 mmHg (0.8 kPa).

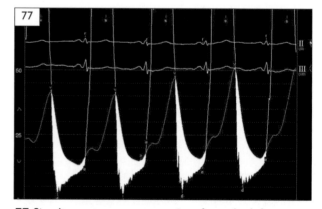

**77** Simultaneous pressure tracings from the left ventricle (yellow) and left atrium (red) from a patient with documented severe mitral stenosis. Note the elevated pulmonary wedge pressure and the transmitral gradient persisting throughout diastole.

fibrillation, systemic embolism (cerebral, coronary, and renal), infective endocarditis, hoarseness secondary to left recurrent laryngeal nerve compression, and right-sided heart failure secondary to severe pulmonary hypertension (Wood, 1954; Chambers, 2001).

SIGNS

Pinkish-purple patches may be present on the cheeks (mitral facies) as a result of the low cardiac output and associated vasoconstriction. Examination of the jugular venous pulsations often reveals a prominent a wave in sinus rhythm and a single giant v wave in atrial fibrillation. With precordial palpation, the examiner may note a diastolic thrill at the apex or a right ventricular lift at the left sternal edge.

Auscultation will demonstrate a loud $S_1$ if the leaflets are pliable. $P_2$ becomes loud with pulmonary hypertension, but later merges with $A_2$ as pulmonary vascular compliance decreases. Pulmonary hypertension may also produce pulmonary artery dilatation with an associated pulmonic ejection sound, a tricuspid regurgitation murmur, a Graham Steell murmur of pulmonic regurgitation, and a right-sided $S_4$. Sudden tensing of the mitral leaflets produces the classic opening snap heard best with the diaphragm at the apex in early diastole. This is generally followed by the low-pitched, apical diastolic rumble characteristic of MS. The duration of the murmur correlates with the severity of obstruction. Palpation of the apical impulse will facilitate auscultation of localized murmurs. 'Silent' MS results from right ventricular hypertrophy with posterior rotation of the left ventricle, such that the rumble is inaudible or heard laterally. Brief exercise may augment the murmur of MS by increasing cardiac output and flow through the valve.

LABORATORY FINDINGS

*Electrocardiography*

Evidence of LA enlargement is found in 90% of patients with significant MS in sinus rhythm (Cooksey *et al.*, 1977; Zeng *et al.*, 2003). With the development of pulmonary hypertension, right ventricular hypertrophy (RVH) is often seen on the electrocardiogram (ECG). As pulmonary artery pressure rises, the mean frontal QRS access generally shifts further rightward, reflecting the development of RVH (Donoso *et al.*, 1957). Some of these findings are presented in **78**.

*Chest radiography*

Left atrial enlargement is commonly seen. Once pulmonary hypertension is established, radiographic evidence of pulmonary artery, right ventricular, and right atrial enlargement may be present. The lung markings may include Kerley A and B lines (**79, 80**).

**78** 12-lead electrocardiogram from a patient with documented mitral stenosis. Note the evidence of right ventricular hypertrophy (right axis deviation and R >S in $V_1$) which often accompanies this valve lesion.

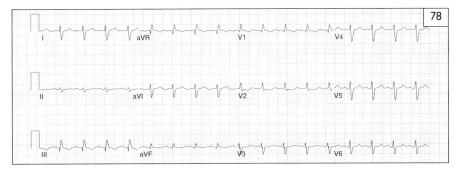

**79, 80** Postero-anterior and lateral chest films of a patient with combined mitral stenosis and mitral regurgitation. Left atrial enlargement is evidenced by the straightening of the left heart border (the loss of the normal concavity). (Courtesy of Bill Black, MD.)

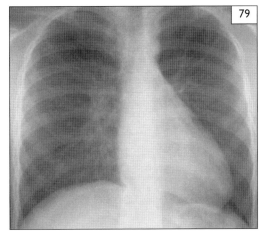
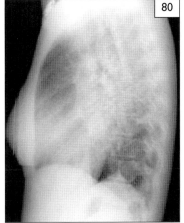

Cardiac catheterization with transatrial septal puncture may allow direct measurement of the mitral pressure gradient, left atrial size, and visualization of thrombi (**81**), but has largely been supplanted by echocardiography (Braunwald, 2001).

*Echocardiography*
Echocardiography is the principal means of assessing MS. 2D findings pertinent in the evaluation of MS include doming of the anterior leaflet, decreased leaflet mobility, increased leaflet calcification and thickness, commissural fusion, calcification of the subvalvular apparatus, and increased LA size (**82, 83**). Doppler interrogation of intracardiac flow allows quantitation of the pressure gradient across the mitral valve, estimation of pulmonary artery systolic pressure, and estimation of the mitral valve area (*Table 16*). The effect of exercise can be assessed by performing the same measurements during supine bicycle exercise or during dobutamine administration.

*Cardiac magnetic resonance*
As in aortic stenosis, cardiac magnetic resonance (CMR) is being increasingly employed in the evaluation of stenotic mitral lesions. As noted in Chapter 4, the high spatial resolution of CMR has been used to measure valve area directly by planimetry. In addition, in the case of MS, velocity encoded CMR has been used to measure pressure half-time, a long-standing Doppler measure of MS. This approach has been recently validated (Lin *et al.*, 2004). Like echo, it carries no risk of ionizing radiation and no risks of iodinated contrast agents such as nephrotoxicity or anaphylaxis. Its advantage over echocardiography is its lack of dependence upon good echocardiographic windows. An important limitation is the contraindication of exposing patients with pacemakers or implantable cardioverter devices (or other ferromagnetic prostheses) to the high magnetic fields used in MR.

**Natural history**
Data on the frequency and rate of progression of MS are very limited. Older studies suggest progression in 32% of patients and stability in the remainder. Among those with progressive stenosis, the mean rate was 0.3 ±0.2 cm²/year (Dubin *et al.*, 1971). In one series, asymptomatic patients had a 10-year survival of 84% but a 20-year survival of only 38% (Rowe *et al.*, 1960). Given the shift from rheumatic heart disease to degenerative etiologies seen in the past 40 years, it is uncertain how generalizable these figures are to patients today. However, for ethical reasons, it is very unlikely that these data will ever be updated.

Atrial fibrillation is a common sequela; it is seen more often in older patients and those with left atrial enlargment, usually begins paroxysmally, is often asymptomatic, and may be accompanied by embolic events, including permanently disabling stroke (Iung *et al.*, 2002).

**Medical management and follow-up**
Avoiding excess physical exertion is recommended in moderate to severe cases to avoid the increased LA pressure associated with an elevated cardiac output and heart rate. Limiting sodium intake or diuretic use may be necessary if pulmonary congestion is present.

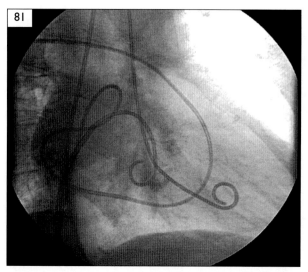

**81** Fluoroscopic image of an invasive hemodynamic assessment of mitral stenosis. Note the presence of a pigtail catheter placed in retrograde fashion in the left ventricle, another pigtail catheter placed through the interatrial septum into the left atrium, and a pulmonary artery catheter looped in the right atrium before passing through the right ventricle and out the pulmonary artery, off the screen into the right lung. (Courtesy of John Robb, MD.)

Rheumatic fever prophylaxis is indicated in patients with rheumatic valve disease. All patients require endocarditis prophylaxis. Negative chronotropic agents are often useful to maximize diastolic filling time. Atrial fibrillation is often poorly tolerated and requires anticoagulation and heart rate control. Hemodynamic instability demands urgent, direct current cardioversion (DCCV). Elective DCCV of a patient in atrial fibrillation of unknown duration or known to have persisted for >48 hours must be preceded by 3 weeks of anticoagulation or by a transesophageal echocardiogram (TEE) to exclude the presence of atrial thrombus. In both strategies, anticoagulation should be continued for at least 4 weeks following cardioversion and indefinitely if atrial fibrillation recurs. Antiarrhythmic agents may be employed in an attempt to maintain sinus rhythm, but should not be expected to provide indefinite success in this.

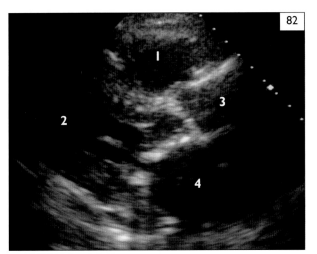

**82** Parasternal long axis echocardiographic view of a patient with mitral stenosis. Note the thickened mitral valve leaflets and their limited excursion. 1: right ventricle; 2: left ventricle; 3: ascending aorta; 4: left atrium.

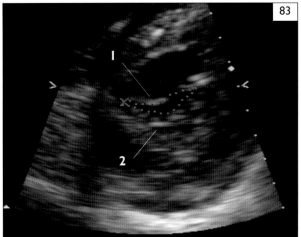

**83** Echocardiographic measurement of the mitral valve orifice by planimetry in a short axis view of the same patient seen in **82**. 1: anterior mitral valve leaflet; 2: posterior mitral valve leaflet.

| **Table 16** Echocardiographic data used to estimate mitral valve area | | | | | | | |
|---|---|---|---|---|---|---|---|
| | **Measure used for calculation** | **Selected measure** | **1** | **2** | **3** | **4** | **5** |
| MV peak V | 272 cm/sec | avg | 281 | 267 | 287 | 273 | 253 |
| MV V$_2$ trace | 11.8 | avg | 12.5 | 12.1 | 13.4 | 12.0 | 8.98 |
| MV dec slope | 501 cm/sec$^2$ | avg | 401 | 472 | 524 | 570 | 535 |
| MV P$^1/_2$t max V | 274 cm/sec | avg | 271 | 267 | 293 | 279 | 259 |
| LVOT diam | 1.83 cm | | 1.83 | | | | |
| MV max PG | 29.6 mmHg (4 kPa) | | MV mean PG | | | 11.8 mmHg (1.6 kPa) | |
| MVA (P$^1/_2$t) | 1.38 cm$^2$ | | | | | | |

LVOT: left ventricular outflow tract; MV: mitral valve; MVA: mitral valve area; P$^1/_2$t: pressure half-time; PG: pressure gradient; V: velocity.

**Table 17** Recommendations for anticoagulation in mitral stenosis

| Indication | Class |
| --- | --- |
| Patients with atrial fibrillation, paroxysmal or chronic | I |
| Patients with a prior embolic event | I |
| Patients with severe MS and left atrial dimension ≥55 mm by echocardiography* | IIb |
| All other patients with MS | III |

MS: mitral stenosis. *Based on grade C recommendation given this indication by the American College of Chest Physicians Fourth Consensus Conference on Antithrombotic Therapy. The Working Group of the European Society of Cardiology uses a lower threshold of left atrial dimension (>50 mm) for recommending anticoagulation. (Adapted from Bonow RO, Carabello B, de Leon AC Jr, *et al.* (1998). ACC/AHA guidelines for the management of patients with valvular heart disease. *Journal of the American College of Cardiology* **32**:1486–1588.)

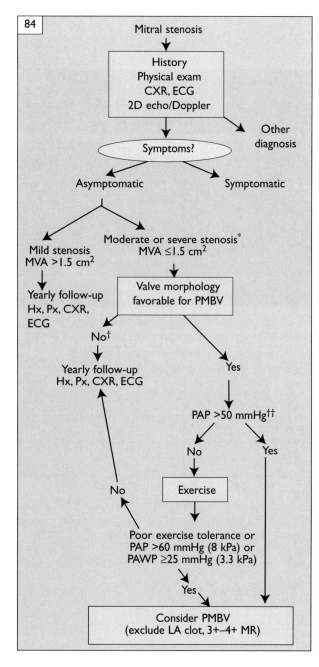

Risk factors for stroke include age, atrial fibrillation, and prior systemic embolism. The severity of obstruction, LA size, and presence of heart failure do not predict embolic events. Although there are no randomized trials addressing this issue, retrospective studies suggest benefit from systemic anticoagulation. The ACC/AHA recommendations are listed in *Table 17*.

Asymptomatic patients should be evaluated annually and sooner if symptoms develop (84).

**Percutaneous intervention**

Percutaneous mitral balloon valvotomy (PMBV) was developed in the mid-1980s. It is considered in patients with suitable anatomy (i.e. pliable leaflets, no commissural fusion, and minimal subvalvular calcification) and contraindications to surgery (Vahanian, 2001).

**84** Management strategy for patients with mitral stenosis. CXR: chest X-ray; ECG: electrocardiogram; Hx: history; LA: left atrium; MR: mitral regurgitation; MVA: mitral valve area; PAP: pulmonary artery pressure; PAWP: pulmonary artery wedge pressure; PMBV: percutaneous mitral balloon valvotomy; Px: physical exam. *The committee recognizes that there may be variability in the measurement of MVA and that the mean transmitral gradient, PAWP, and PAP should also be taken into consideration. †There is controversy as to whether patients with severe mitral stenosis (MVA <1.0 cm²) and severe pulmonary hypertension (PAP >60–80 mmHg [8–10.7 kPa]) should undergo mitral valve replacement to prevent right ventricular failure. ††Assuming no other cause for pulmonary hypertension is present. (Adapted from Bonow RO, Carabello B, de Leon AC Jr, *et al.* (1998) ACC/AHA guidelines for the management of patients with valvular heart disease. *Journal of the American College of Cardiology* **32**:1486–1588.)

The procedure is performed with an hour glass-shaped balloon (Inoue balloon) using a trans-septal approach (85). Considerable experience is required to perform it well. Randomized trials of patients ideally suited to PMBV suggest that percutaneous intervention yields results superior to closed commissurotomy and equal to open commissurotomy (Cardoso *et al*., 2002). Valve area usually doubles with an accompanying 50–60% decrease in transmitral gradient. Contra-indications include unfavorable valve morphology (see above), 3–4+ mitral regurgitation (MR), and LA thrombus. Well-selected patients in experienced centers have procedural mortality rates of <1%. In a contemporary European series of 492 consecutive patients with severe MS in functional class I or II, there were no procedural related deaths or embolism and a 2% rate of severe MR. Nine years post procedure, 77% remained asymptomatic (Iung *et al*., 1998). In addition to severe MR, other possible complications include a large residual atrioseptal defect, left ventricular perforation, embolic events, and myocardial infarction (Bonow *et al*., 1998). The ACC/AHA guidelines for PMBV are shown in *Table 18*. Citing the relative safety of the procedure, the favorable functional outcomes compared to historical controls, and a decreased risk of thromboembolic events, the European Society of Cardiology Working Group proposes that percutaneous intervention be considered in asymptomatic patients with severe MS (i.e. mitral valve area <1 $cm^2/m^2$) with an increased risk of embolism (prior emboli, dense spontaneous echo contrast in the LA on TEE, or recent paroxysmal atrial fibrillation [PAF]) or hemodynamic decompensation (pulmonary artery systolic pressure >50 mmHg [6.7 kPa] at rest or >60 mmHg [8 kPa] with exercise, planned pregnancy, or need for major surgery). A notable trans-Atlantic difference in guidelines is the greater use of body surface area (BSA) adjusted valve area criteria in Europe (Iung *et al*., 2002).

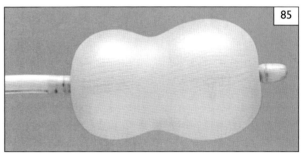

**85** Inoue balloon catheter used for percutaneous valvuloplasty. (Courtesy of Toray Industries (America), Inc.)

**Table 18** Recommendations for percutaneous mitral balloon valvotomy

| Indication | Class |
| --- | --- |
| Symptomatic patients (NYHA functional Class II, III or IV), moderate or severe MS (MVA =1.5 $cm^2$)*, and valve morphology favorable for percutaneous balloon valvotomy in the absence of left atrial thrombus or moderate to severe MR | I |
| Asymptomatic patients with moderate or severe MS (MVA =1.5 $cm^2$)*, and valve morphology favorable for percutaneous ballon valvotomy who have pulmonary hypertension (pulmonary artery systolic pressure >50 mmHg [6.7 kPa] at rest or 60 mmHg [8 kPa] with exercise) in the absence of left atrial thrombus or moderate to severe MR | IIa |
| Patients with NYHA functional Class III–IV symptoms, moderate or severe MS (MVA =1.5 $cm^2$)*, and a nonpliable calcified valve who are at high risk for surgery in the absence of left atrial thrombus or moderate to severe MR | IIa |
| Asymptomatic patients, moderate or severe MS (MVA =1.5 $cm^2$)*, and valve morphology favorable for percutaneous balloon valvotomy who have new onset of atrial fibrillation in the absence of left atrial thrombus or moderate to severe MR | IIb |
| Patients in NYHA functional Class III–IV, moderate or severe MS (MVA =1.5 $cm^2$)*, and a nonpliable calcified valve who are low-risk candidates for surgery | IIb |
| Patients with mild MS | III |

MR: mitral regurgitation; MS: mitral stenosis; MVA: mitral valve area; NYHA: New York Heart Association. * The committee recognizes that there may be variability in the measurement of mitral valve area and that the mean transmitral gradient, pulmonary artery wedge pressure, and pulmonary artery pressure at rest or during exercise should also be taken into consideration. (Adapted from Bonow RO, Carabello B, de Leon AC Jr, *et al*. (1998). ACC/AHA guidelines for the management of patients with valvular heart disease. *Journal of the American College of Cardiology* **32**:1486–1588.)

Symptomatic patients with a mitral valve area (MVA) <1.5 cm$^2$ or a mean gradient >5 mmHg (0.7 kPa) should be considered for intervention. If a patient appears to have class III or IV symptoms but does not meet the above criteria, echocardiography or cardiac catheterization during exercise can be used to assess the impact of increasing heart rate and cardiac output. Those patients with elevation of the mean gradient beyond 15 mmHg (2 kPa), pulmonary artery systemic pressure >60 mmHg (8 kPa), or pulmonary capillary wedge pressure >25 mmHg (3.3 kPa) are generally considered for intervention depending on their overall health status (Bonow *et al.*, 1998). This approach is outlined in **86** and **87**. European guidelines

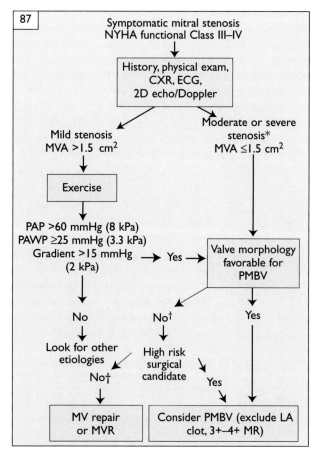

**86** Management strategy for patients with mitral stenosis and mild symptoms. CXR: chest X-ray; ECG: electrocardiogram; LA: left atrium; MR: mitral regurgitation; MVA: mitral valve area; PAP: pulmonary artery pressure; PAWP: pulmonary artery wedge pressure; PMBV: percutaneous mitral balloon valvotomy. *The committee recognizes that there may be variability in the measurement of MVA and that the mean transmitral gradient, PAWP, and PAP should also be taken into consideration.†There is controversy as to whether patients with severe mitral stenosis (MVA <1.0 cm$^2$) and severe pulmonary hypertension (PAP >60–80 mmHg [8–10.7 kPa]) should undergo mitral valve replacement to prevent right ventricular failure. (Adapted from Bonow RO, Carabello B, de Leon AC Jr, *et al.* (1998). ACC/AHA guidelines for the management of patients with valvular heart disease. *Journal of the American College of Cardiology* **32**:1486–1588.)

**87** Management strategy for patients with mitral stenosis and moderate to severe symptoms. CXR: chest X-ray; ECG: electrocardiogram; LA: left atrium; MR: mitral regurgitation; MV: mitral valve; MVA: mitral valve area; MVR: mitral valve replacement; NYHA: New York Heart Association; PAP: pulmonary artery pressure; PAWP: pulmonary artery wedge pressure; PMBV: percutaneous mitral balloon valvotomy. *The committee recognizes that there may be variability in the measurement of MVA and that the mean transmitral gradient, PAWP, and PAP should also be taken into consideration.†It is controversial as to which patients with less favorable valve morphology should undergo PMBV rather than MV surgery. (Adapted from Bonow RO, Carabello B, de Leon AC Jr, *et al.* (1998). ACC/AHA guidelines for the management of patients with valvular heart disease. *Journal of the American College of Cardiology* **32**:1486–1588.)

are similar, with recommendations that percutaneous intervention be considered for all patients with symptomatic mitral stenosis who lack the same contraindications cited above (Prendergast *et al.*, 1996).

## Surgical intervention

### SURGICAL COMMISSUROTOMY

While first proposed in 1902, mitral commissurotomy was not successfully performed until the 1920s. The implementation of cardiopulmonary bypass in the 1960s permitted surgeons to shift from closed commissurotomies to open approaches for repair and valve replacement. Resection of the thrombus-prone LA appendage is sometimes performed as an adjunct to mitral valve surgery. Operative mortality in large centers ranges from 1 to 3%, with 5-year complication-free survival rates of 80–90% (Bonow *et al.*, 1998).

### MITRAL VALVE REPAIR AND REPLACEMENT

When patients not suitable for valvotomy progress to class III or class IV symptoms, their poor prognosis with medical therapy mandates consideration of valve surgery. When technically feasible, repair is preferred over replacement because it does not include the risk of the anticoagulation required in mechanical valves and the risk of structural failure present in both tissue and mechanical prostheses. The ACC/AHA guidelines for surgical referral are listed in *Tables 19* and *20*. Operative mortality rates range from 5 to 20% depending on patient factors and the experience of the surgical team. Possible complications include valve thrombus with embolism as well as prosthetic valve endocarditis with subsequent dehiscence of the prosthesis. Symptom improvement is generally immediate. Following both surgical and percutaneous intervention, patients require continued follow-up to monitor for recurrent symptoms and infective endocarditis prophylaxis.

**Table 19** Recommendations for mitral valve repair for mitral stenosis

| Indication | Class |
|---|---|
| Patients with NYHA functional Class III–IV symptoms, moderate or severe MS (MVA =1.5 cm$^2$)*, and valve morphology favorable for repair if percutaneous mitral balloon valvotomy is not available | I |
| Patients with NYHA functional Class III–IV symptoms, moderate or severe MS (MVA =1.5cm$^2$)*, and valve morphology favorable for repair if a left atrial thrombus is present despite anticoagulation | I |
| Patients with NYHA functional Class III–IV symptoms, moderate or severe MS (MVA =1.5 cm$^2$)*, and a nonpliable or calcified valve with the decision to proceed with either repair or replacement made at the time of the operation | I |
| Patients in NYHA functional Class I, moderate or severe MS (MVA =1.5 cm$^2$)*, and valve morphology favorable for repair who have had recurrent episodes of embolic events on adequate anticoagulation | IIb |
| Patients with NYHA functional Class I–IV symptoms, and mild MS | III |

MS: mitral stenosis; MVA: mitral valve area; NYHA: New York Heart Association. *The committee recognizes that there may be variability in the measurement of mitral valve area and that the mean transmitral gradient, pulmonary artery wedge pressure, and pulmonary artery pressure at rest or during exercise should also be considered. (Adapted from Bonow RO, Carabello B, de Leon AC Jr, *et al.* (1998). ACC/AHA guidelines for the management of patients with valvular heart disease. *Journal of the American College of Cardiology* **32**:1486–1588.)

**Table 20** Recommendations for mitral valve replacement for mitral stenosis

| Indication | Class |
|---|---|
| Patients with moderate or severe MS (MVA =1.5 cm$^2$)* and NYHA functional Class III–IV symptoms who are not considered candidates for percutaneous balloon valvotomy or mitral valve repair | I |
| Patients with severe MS (MVA = 1 cm$^2$)*, and severe pulmonary hypertension (pulmonary artery systolic pressure >60–80 mmHg [8–10.7 kPa]) with NYHA functional Class I–II symptoms who are not considered candidates for percutaneous balloon valvotomy or mitral valve repair | IIa |

MS: mitral stenosis; MVA: mitral valve area; NYHA: New York Heart Association. *The committee recognizes that there may be variability in the measurement of mitral valve area and that the mean transmitral gradient, pulmonary artery wedge pressure, and pulmonary artery pressure should also be considered. (Adapted from Bonow RO, Carabello B, de Leon AC Jr, *et al.* (1998). ACC/AHA guidelines for the management of patients with valvular heart disease. *Journal of the American College of Cardiology* **32**:1486–1588.)

## Case study

A 37-year-old woman presented to the occupational health nurse with a concern of recurrent respiratory infections, trouble breathing when she lay down at night, and new vocal hoarseness. These problems had developed slowly over the past 3–4 months. Her review of systems was remarkable for a change in her voice (hoarse), fatigue, and breathlessness with activity over the past year. She had delayed seeking medical attention for her symptoms because she feared it might jeopardize her employment.

Her past medical history was remarkable for rheumatic fever as a child, fibrocystic breast disease, and primary hypothyroidism. Her only medications were levothyroxine and calcium supplements.

She was employed as an electrical engineer by a large manufacturing concern in the southeastern US. Born and raised in Pakistan, she was now married with two young children. She had never smoked and consumed no alcohol. There was no family history of premature cardiopulmonary disease.

Initially concerned about possible occupational airborn irritants, the nurse referred her to the occupational health physician at the plant. Her exam was remarkable for a blood pressure of 122/54 mmHg (16.3/7.2 kPa) in the right arm and 126/50 mmHg (16.8/6.7 kPa) in the left arm. Pulse was 94 bpm and irregularly irregular. She had ruddy cheeks and cool extremities. There were wet crackles extending 1/4 up both lung fields. Her estimated right atrial pressure was 15 cm of $H_2O$ and abdominojugular reflux was present. She had an RV heave. Her point of maximal intensity (PMI) was not displaced and was of normal size and duration. $P_2$ was loud. A high-pitched, extra heart sound was heard in early diastole at the lower left sternal border and a low pitched rumble extending throughout the remainder of diastole was heard at the apex. The murmur clearly increased in volume after 10 steps up and down the exam table step. She had 1+ lower extremity edema. She was begun on metoprolol, furosemide, and warfarin as an outpatient that day, with follow-up in 5 days.

An echocardiogram performed 2 weeks later revealed severe MS with a mean pressure gradient estimated by Doppler interrogation of 18 mmHg (2.4 kPa). The estimated mitral valve area was 0.9 cm$^2$. There was thickening of the leaflets with reduced excursion and moderate fibrosis of the subvalvular apparatus (the chordae and papillary muscles). There was no calcification of the valve. The left atrium was severely enlarged. Based on intracardiac flow velocities, the estimated pulmonary artery pressure was 70/40 mmHg (9.3/5.3 kPa). Moderate right atrial enlargement was seen. Left ventricular function was normal.

After consultation with an interventional cardiologist with extensive experience in percutaneous mitral balloon valvulotomy, she was admitted to the hospital in the morning and underwent transesophageal echocardiography that confirmed MS and revealed mild MR and no evidence of atrial thrombus. She then underwent placement of a PA catheter revealing a mean pulmonary capillary wedge pressure (PCWP) of 36 mmHg (4.8 kPa) with a v wave of 50 mmHg (6.7 kPa). Following this, she underwent passage of a guidewire across the intra-atrial septum, followed by positioning of an hourglass-shaped balloon and mitral valvotomy. Immediately following the procedure her PCWP was 20 mmHg (2.7 kPa), her pulmonary artery systolic pressure had dropped to 45 mmHg (6.0 kPa) and her invasively measured mean transmitral pressure gradient had fallen to 7 mmHg (0.9 kPa).

One week post procedure she was back at work. One year later she was still in atrial fibrillation, but was in NYHA functional class I.

## COMMENTS

This case highlights the symptoms and findings of severe rheumatic MS, the common echo findings and hemodynamic findings typical of severe disease. She met all the usual thresholds for intervention. The role of medications was to control heart rate, decongest the lungs, and protect against stroke. Her valve morphology and function (absence of severe fibrosis, heavy calcification, moderate or severe MR) allowed her to be considered for PMBV. She fortunately had a good result.

## References

Bonow RO, Carabello B, de Leon AC Jr, *et al.* (1998). ACC/AHA guidelines for the management of patients with valvular heart disease: a report of the American College of Cardiology/American Heart Association Task Force on Practice Guidelines (Committee on Management of Patients with Valvular Heart Disease). *Journal of the American College of Cardiology* **32**:1486–1588.

Braunwald E (2001). Valvular heart disease. In: *Heart Disease: A Textbook of Cardiovascular Medicine.* E Braunwald, DP Zipes, P Libby (eds). WB Saunders, Philadelphia, ch 46, pp.1643–1722.

Cardoso LF, Grinberg M, Rati MA, *et al.* (2002). Comparison between percutaneous balloon valvuloplasty and open commissurotomy for mitral stenosis. A prospective and randomized study. *Cardiology* **98**(4):186–190.

Chambers J (2001). The clinical and diagnostic features of mitral valve disease. *Hospital Medicine (London)* **62**(2):72–78.

Cooksey JD, Dunn M, Massie E (1977). *Clinical Vectorcardiography and Electrocardiography*, 2nd edn. Year Book Medical Publishers, Chicago, p. 272.

Donoso E, Jick S, Braunwald E, *et al.* (1957). The spatial vectorcardiogram in mitral valve disease. *American Heart Journal* **53**:760.

Dubin AA, March HW, Chon K, Selzer A (1971). Longitudinal hemodynamic and clinical study of mitral stenosis. *Circulation* **44**:381–389.

Iung B, Garbarz E, Helou S, *et al.* (1998). What are the results of percutaneous mitral commissurotomy in patients with few or no symptoms? (Abstract). *European Heart Journal* **19**(Abstract Supplement):529.

Iung B, Gohlke-Bärwolf, Tornos P, *et al.* on behalf of the Working Group on Valvular Heart Disease (2002). Recommendations on the management of the asymptomatic patient with valvular heart disease. *European Heart Journal* **23**(16):1253–1266.

Lin SJ, Brown PA, Watkins MP, *et al.* (2004). Quantification of stenotic mitral valve area with magnetic resonance imaging and comparison with Doppler ultrasound. *Journal of the American College of Cardiology* **44**(1):133–137.

Prendergast B, Banning AP, Hall RJC (1996). Valvular heart disease: recommendations for investigation and management. Summary of guidelines produced by a working group of the British Cardiac Society and the Research Unit of the Royal College of Physicians. *Journal of the Royal College of Physicians of London* **30**:309–315.

Roberts WC, Perloff JK (1972). Mitral valvular disease: a clinicopathologic survey of the conditions causing the mitral valve to function abnormally. *Annals of Internal Medicine* **77**:939–975.

Rowe JC, Bland EF, Sprague HB, White PD (1960). The course of mitral stenosis without surgery: ten and twenty-year perspectives. *Annals of Internal Medicine* **52**: 741–749.

Vahanian A (2001). Balloon valvuloplasty. *Heart* **85**(2):223–228.

Wood P (1954). An appreciation of mitral stenosis. *British Medical Journal* **1**:1051–1063.

Zeng C, Wei T, Zhao R, Wang C, Chen L, Wang L (2003). Electrocardiographic diagnosis of left atrial enlargement in patients with mitral stenosis: the value of the P-wave area. *Acta Cardiologica* **58**(2):139–141.

# Chapter Eight

# Mitral Valve Prolapse

## Definition

Mitral valve prolapse (MVP) has been a controversial topic in valvular heart disease. The current definition, as outlined by the ACC/AHA task force, includes echocardiographic findings of atrial displacement of mitral leaflets, accompanied by auscultatory findings of a midsystolic click. It is the most prevalent of valvular heart diseases, affecting between 2% and 6% of the population, and is the most common cause of mitral regurgitation (Bonow *et al.*, 1998).

One popular classification system distinguishes primary MVP from secondary causes of MVP. Primary MVP is characterized by pathologic abnormalities of the mitral valve itself. Secondary MVP refers to conditions in which the principal abnormality lies in the supporting apparatus.

Patients who have only mild echocardiographic prolapse without associated morphologic or auscultatory findings are not considered to have this syndrome (O'Rourke, 1996; Levine *et al.*, 1982).

## Etiology

In primary MVP, the histologic appearance of the leaflets is notable for a dramatic increase in the volume of the spongiosa, the layer sandwiched between the atrialis and the ventricularis collagen-rich surfaces (88). The myxomatous proliferation of the spongiosa results in the gross features of leaflet fibrosis and redundancy, with leaflet thickness exceeding 5 mm and elongation of the chordae tendonae (Lucas and Edwards, 1982). The tricuspid valve is similarly affected in 40% of patients. Epidemiologically, the condition may appear as an isolated case, inherited in

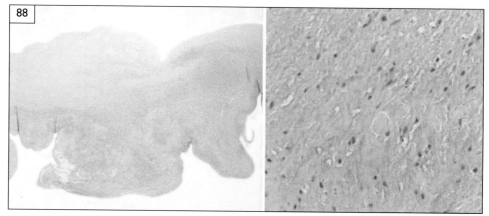

**88** Photomicrograph of a myxomatous mitral valve. Note the thickened and redundant nature of the valve. (Courtesy of Nora Ratcliff, MD.)

an autosomal dominant fashion, or linked to a connective tissue disease. Some investigators have suggested an underlying defect in mesenchymal cell lines. Supporting this hypothesis is the clinical association with the skeletal abnormalities of Marfan's syndrome, straight back syndrome, pectus excavatum, von Willebrand disease, and primary hypomastia (Rosenberg *et al.*, 1983). Other associated conditions include secundum atrial-septal defects (ASDs) and left-sided atrioventricular bypass tracts with Wolff–Parkinson–White (WPW) syndrome. More likely a result than a cause, autonomic nervous system overactivity has been identified in patients with symptomatic MVP (Gaffney *et al.*, 1983).

Secondary MVP occurs when there is distortion of the mitral valve supporting apparatus (i.e. annulus, chordae, papillary muscles, and left ventricular [LV] walls). This occurs in diverse conditions including ischemic heart disease, rheumatic heart disease, and conditions of decreased LV volume arising from dehydration, ASD, hypertropic cardiomyopathy, and pulmonary hypertension.

## Clinical presentation

In many patients, the diagnosis is made incidentally in the course of a physical exam or an echocardiogram performed for an unrelated reason. Other patients present with symptoms which appear related to the underlying valve pathology. These include atypical chest pain, palpitations unaccompanied by arrhythmias on Holter monitor, dyspnea, fatigue, anxiety, and transient ischemic attacks (TIAs).

Physical exam is the foundation of evaluation. The characteristic finding is one or more short, high-pitched, midsystolic clicks, a result of the mitral valve apparatus abruptly drawing taut as the leaflets prolapse into the left atrium. Dynamic auscultation (the use of maneuvers to alter a murmur) may confirm the findings. By reducing end-diastolic volume, standing hastens prolapse and moves the click closer to $S_1$. Conversely, squatting delays prolapse by increasing LV filling and hence moves the click closer to $S_2$.

The electrocardiogram (ECG) is usually normal, but may demonstrate nonspecific ST-T wave abnormalities, u waves, or a prolonged QT interval. Ambulatory ECG monitoring is not indicated in asymptomatic patients but may be useful in patients who complain of palpitations. Often, no arrhythmias are found during symptoms. In the absence of severe mitral regurgitation (MR) or Marfan's syndrome, chest radiographs add little to the evaluation (Bonow *et al.*, 1998).

Echocardiography is the principal means of confirming the diagnosis. In 1986, diagnostic criteria based on auscultation and echocardiography were published (Perloff *et al.*, 1986) (*Table 21*). In this scheme, only the presence of one or more major criteria established the diagnosis. A recent consensus

---

**Table 21** Diagnostic criteria in mitral valve prolapse

| Major criteria | Minor criteria |
|---|---|
| **Auscultation** | **Auscultation** |
| Mid- to late systolic clicks and late systolic murmur 'whoop' alone in combination at the cardiac apex | Loud $S_1$ with an apical holosystolic murmur |
| **2D echocardiogram** | **2D echocardiogram** |
| Marked superior systolic displacement of mitral leaflets (2 mm above annulus) with coaptation point at or superior to annular plane | Isolated mild to moderate superior systolic displacement of posterior mitral leaflet |
| Mild to moderate superior systolic displacement of mitral leaflets with: | Moderate superior systolic displacement of both mitral leaflets |
|     Chordal rupture | **Echocardiogram plus history of:** |
|     Doppler mitral regurgitation | Mild to moderate superior systolic displacement of mitral leaflets with: |
|     Annular dilatation |     Focal neurologic attacks or amaurosis fugax in the young patient |
| **Echocardiogram plus auscultation** |     First-degree relatives with major criteria |
| Mild to moderate superior systolic displacement of mitral leaflets with: | |
|     Prominent mid- to late systolic clicks at the cardiac apex | (Adapted from Perloff JK, Child JS, Edwards JE (1986). New guidelines for the clinical diagnosis of mitral valve prolapse. *American Journal of Cardiology* **57**:1124–1129.) |
|     Apical late systolic or holosystolic murmur in the young patient | |
|     Late systolic 'whoop' | |

document urged the inclusion of abnormal valve morphology in addition to prolapse. These structural changes may include leaflet thickening, redundancy, annular dilatation, and chordal elongation. Doppler echocardiography is useful in identifying and quantifying associated MR (Bonow *et al.*, 1998). Examples of echocardiographic images of a patient with MVP are presented in **89–92**.

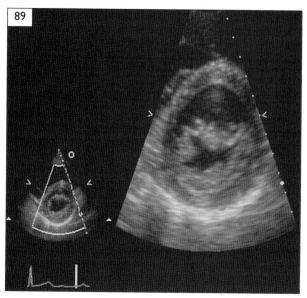

**89** Parasternal short axis echocardiographic view of a myxomatous mitral valve. Note the redundant (wavy) and thickened leaflets.

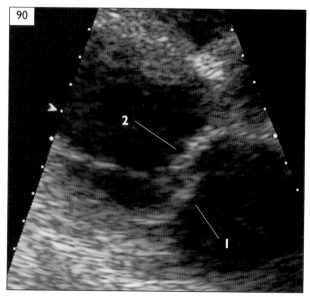

**90** Magnified parasternal long axis echocardiographic image of the mitral valve showing prolapse of the posterior mitral valve leaflet (1). Note the thickening characteristic of myxomatous valve leaflets. 2: anterior mitral valve leaflet.

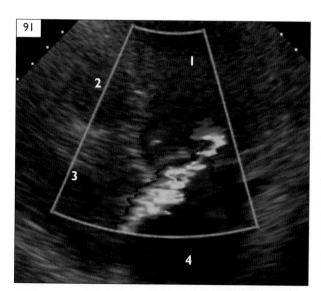

**91** Magnified apical 4-chamber echocardiographic image of the mitral valve showing prolapse of the posterior mitral valve leaflet. 1: left ventricle; 2: right ventricle; 3: right atrium; 4: left atrium.

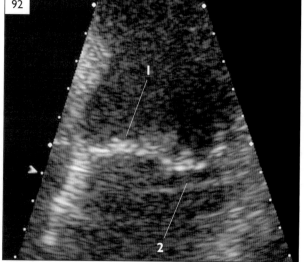

**92** Color flow Doppler imaging of the same patient as **91** demonstrating the anteriorly directed regurgitant jet resulting from the posterior leaflet prolapse. 1: anterior mitral valve leaflet; 2: posterior mitral valve leaflet.

## Natural history

The natural history is usually benign; there is no increase in age-adjusted mortality (Devereux *et al.*, 1982; Freed *et al.*, 2002). However, there are exceptions. Some individuals develop progressive MR accompanied by left atrial dilatation, atrial fibrillation and, in severe cases, left ventricular dilatation, pulmonary hypertension, and right ventricular failure (Aviernos *et al.*, 2002). Sudden death is rare with a lifetime incidence of <2%, but it may be more likely in familial forms of MVP (Fontana *et al.*, 1991). Infective endocarditis is a very rare complication, but given the prevalence of MVP, this valvular abnormality is the most common underlying abnormality in infective endocarditis. Cerebral events have been attributed to embolization of MVP-related fibrin (Wilson *et al.*, 1977).

## Medical management

Asymptomatic patients with no significant MR should be evaluated every 3–5 years. Moderate to severe MR or a change in symptoms should prompt more frequent follow-up.

Alcohol, caffeine, and cigarettes should be avoided by patients suffering from palpitations. Exercise limitations are indicated only in patients with left ventricular dilatation, left ventricular systolic dysfunction, uncontrolled tachyarrhythmias, long QT syndrome, family history of sudden death, or aortic root dilatation (Fontana *et al.*, 1991).

Aspirin is recommended in those patients with TIAs but no evidence of atrial fibrillation. Coumadin therapy should be instituted if patients with MVP have had prior strokes or have recurrent TIAs despite aspirin. Beta-blockers may be useful in those patients whose symptoms persist after elimination of stimulants. Patients with MVP and a regurgitant murmur or clearly abnormal valve morphology should receive endocarditis prophylaxis.

## Surgical intervention

The indications for mitral valve surgery are the same as for other causes of MR. These are outlined in Chapter 9 but include LV dilatation, LV systolic dysfunction, atrial fibrillation, and pulmonary hypertension. Currently, the preferred surgical approach is repair of the valve, rather than replacement. Usually, this avoids the need for long-term warfarin therapy (Bonow *et al.*, 1998).

## Case study

A 28-year-old waitress visited a cardiologist at the request of her mother who had recently been diagnosed with severe MR and was undergoing mitral valve repair at a nearby medical center. Her mother wanted to make sure that her valve condition had not been inherited by her children. The patient had no physical complaints. She worked 60 hours per week and sang in a country music band. She enjoyed dancing and roller skating and felt she had no trouble keeping up with her peers. She denied palpitations, unusual shortness of breath, trouble sleeping when lying down, and ankle edema. Her medical history was notable for mild asthma and one prior episode of kidney stones. She used an albuterol inhaler less than once per month.

On exam, she was 1.79 m ( 5' 10") with a weight of 58 kg (130 lb). She looked very fit and was in no distress. Her blood pressure was 118/58 mmHg (15.7/7.7 kPa) and her pulse was 66 bpm and regular. Her skin was warm and dry. Thyroid was normal on palpation. Chest exam revealed good air movement bilaterally without crackles or wheezes. Her jugular venous pulsations were normal with an estimated mean right atrial pressure of 6 cm $H_2O$. She had no carotid bruits, no right ventricular heave, and no thrills. Her point of maximal intensity (PMI) was normal and located in the mid clavicular line in the 5th intercostal space. She had a normal $S_1$ and physiologically split $S_2$, with a high-pitched extra heart sound in midsystole, heard best at the apex. There was no murmur. Standing caused the clicking to move closer to $S_1$ and squatting caused it to move closer to $S_2$. The remainder of her exam was normal. Her ECG was normal. She was reassured that she was healthy and no limits were placed on her activity. No prescriptions were given.

Five years later, during her first pregnancy, she was noted to have a 2/6 flow murmur. The midsystolic click had not changed. She had an uneventful delivery after which her murmur disappeared. Ten years later, at age 43 years, she saw a physician as part of an application for additional life insurance. In addition to her midsystolic click she was now noted to have a blowing late systolic murmur, heard best at the apex and radiating to the left upper chest. $P_2$ was not loud and there was no $S_3$. She continued to be very physically active and had no cardiovascular-related complaints. Amoxicillin (2 g 1 hr prior to dental work) was prescribed.

Eight years later, at age 51 years, she was still touring internationally with her band, recording albums, and worked out daily in a spinning (stationary bicycle) class. She felt great. Her exam had not changed. An echocardiogram was performed which showed thickened and redundant mitral valve leaflets, with prolapse of the middle scallop of the posterior leaflet and an anteriorly directed jet of MR. The MR was graded as mild. The left atrium was normal in size. Estimated pulmonary artery systolic pressure was 32 mmHg (4.3 kPa). The tricuspid valve was similarly, but less severely, affected.

COMMENTS

This case demonstrates the typically asymptomatic and benign nature of MVP, the need for infective endocarditis prophylaxis when a murmur is present, the lack of need to proscribe physical activity, and the typical echocardiographic findings.

**References**

Aviernos JF, Gersh BJ, Melton LJ, *et al.* (2002). Natural history of asymptomatic mitral valve prolapse in the community. *Circulation* 106:1355–1361.

Bonow RO, Carabello B, de Leon AC Jr, *et al.* (1998). ACC/AHA guidelines for the management of patients with valvular heart disease: a report of the American College of Cardiology/American Heart Association Task Force on Practice Guidelines (Committee on Management of Patients with Valvular Heart Disease). *Journal of the American College of Cardiology* 32:1486–1588.

Devereux RB, Brown WT, Kramer-Fox R, Sachs I (1982). Inheritance of mitral valve prolapse: effect of age and sex on gene expression. *Annals of Internal Medicine* 97:826–832.

Fontana ME, Sparks EA, Boudoulas H, Wooley CF (1991). Mitral valve prolapse and the mitral valve prolapse syndrome. *Current Problems in Cardiology* 16:309–375.

Freed LA, Benjamin EJ, Levy D, *et al.* (2002). Mitral valve prolapse in the general population: the benign nature of echocardiographic features in the Framingham Heart Study. *Journal of the American College of Cardiology* 40(7):1298–1304.

Gaffney FA, Bastian BC, Lane LB, *et al.* (1983). Abnormal cardiovascular regulation in the mitral valve prolapse syndrome. *American Journal of Cardiology* 52: 316–320.

Levine HJ, Isner JM, Salem DN (1982). Primary versus secondary mitral valve prolapse: clinical features and implications. *Clinical Cardiology* 5:371–375.

Lucas RV Jr, Edwards JE (1982). The floppy mitral valve. *Current Problems in Cardiology* 7:1–48.

O'Rourke RA (1996). The mitral valve prolapse syndrome. In: *Classic Teachings in Clinical Cardiology: A Tribute to W Proctor Harvey MD.* MA Chizner (ed). Laennec, Cedar Grove, New Jersey, pp. 1049–1070.

Perloff JK, Child JS, Edwards JE (1986). New guidelines for the clinical diagnosis of mitral valve prolapse. *American Journal of Cardiology* 57:1124–1129.

Rosenberg CA, Derman GH, Grabb WC, Buda AJ (1983). Hypomastia and mitral valve prolapse: evidence of a linked embryologic and mesenchymal dysplasia. *New England Journal of Medicine* 309:1230–1232.

Wilson LA, Keeling PW, Malcom AD, Russel RW, Webb-Peploe MM (1977). Visual complications of mitral valve prolapse. *British Medical Journal* 2:86–88.

# Chapter Nine

# Chronic Mitral Regurgitation

## Definition

Mitral regurgitation (MR) refers to retrograde flow through the mitral valve during ventricular systole. Among valvular heart diagnoses, it ranks second (after aortic stenosis [AS]) in prevalence (Iung *et al.*, 2002). The severity of MR is usually scored on a 6-point scale, ranging from the physiologic levels of 'none' and 'trace' to pathologic levels 1–4. Both angiographic and echocardiographic means of quantitating regurgitant flow exist. As a noninvasive and contrast-free technique, echocardiographic assessment is the current dominant technology. The variety of subjective and objective criteria used to grade valve regurgitation is beyond the scope of this book, but may be found in echocardiography and angiography texts. When clinical management demands more precise grading of mitral regurgitation, quantitative methods based on careful 2D and Doppler echocardiographic measurements can be employed. These volumetric assessments yield descriptions of severity in terms of effective regurgitant orifice (ERO) and regurgitant stroke volume (RSV). Using this volumetric grading scheme, severe (4+) MR is defined as an ERO exceeding 40 mm$^2$ or a regurgitant volume >60 ml/beat (Tribouilloy *et al.*, 2002).

In addition to severity, MR is classified as acute or chronic. As a result of the sudden volume load imposed on the left ventricle (LV), acute MR is generally a medical emergency with a dramatic presentation and demands urgent attention. Conversely, chronic MR typically has a long asymptomatic phase and requires more careful consideration of management options. Because of the differences in presentation and management, these two entities are treated separately. Acute MR is the focus of Chapter 10.

## Etiology

A common and practical classification scheme is to divide causes of chronic MR into functional (i.e. due to disease extrinsic to the valve) and organic (i.e. due to disruption or deformity of the valve itself) etiologies. Organic causes can be further divided into congenital or acquired.

Functional MR is a common sequela of LV systolic dysfunction. Without aggressive medical intervention, the neurohormonal activation, myocyte loss, and local hemodynamics which accompany poor systolic function conspire to produce LV dilatation and spherical remodeling. Details pertaining to mitral valve function include annular dilatation, diminished mitral annular systolic contraction, and malalignment of the papillary muscles. Together, these changes result in failure of the mitral leaflets to coapt in systole (Trichon and O'Connor, 2002). A recent review of 1421 consecutive patients seen at a referral center with LV ejection fraction (EF) <0.35 revealed an 18.9% prevalence of severe MR and a 29.7% prevalence of moderate MR (48.6% of either grade) (Koelling *et al.*, 2002).

In addition, severe, but transient functional MR may result from ischemic papillary muscle dysfunction. In this case, abnormal relaxation and contraction of the papillary muscle or the LV wall segment to which it attaches may be impaired by ischemia. As a consequence, the valve leaflets do not coapt properly and MR results. This can be challenging to diagnose, since physical exam and echocardiography at rest may be normal. Stress echocardiography is often the best means of making this diagnosis. It is important because revascularization may eradicate the MR. Other functional causes include severe hypertension and extrinsic volume overload.

Organic MR is usually the result of congenital or slowly progressive processes such as mitral valve prolapse, abnormal connective tissue, rheumatic disease or, rarely, medication use. While once common, rheumatic disease has largely been supplanted by degenerative disease as the most common cause of organic MR (**93, 94**).

## Pathophysiology and natural history

The gradual development of increasing regurgitant flow allows time for cardiac adaptation. This includes dilatation of the LV by eccentric hypertrophy, the process of adding sarcomeres in series (Grossman *et al.*, 1975). By this increase in end-diastolic volume, a greater total stroke volume (TSV) is achieved, hence allowing maintenance of normal forward stroke volume (FSV) after deducting the regurgitant stroke volume (RSV), since FSV = TSV – RSV. The left atrium (LA) also enlarges to accept the increased volume at a lower pressure.

However, in the face of increasing regurgitant volume over a period of many years, systolic function may fail resulting in severe LV dilatation, decreased EF, and pulmonary hypertension. LA dilatation predisposes to atrial fibrillation (**95**). If allowed to persist, this phase of decompensation becomes irreversible (Bonow *et al.*, 1998).

Among patients with MR due to flail leaflets, the natural history of patients includes not only the risk of LV dysfunction. In a series comprised mostly of patients in functional classes I and II (71%), the linear mortality rate was 6.3% with a 10-year incidence of heart failure and atrial fibrillation of 63% and 30%, respectively (Ling *et al.*, 1996). Furthermore, the linear rate of sudden cardiac death in this population was 1.8%/year (Grigioni *et al.*, 1999).

## Clinical presentation

### SYMPTOMS

As has been mentioned in reference to other valvular lesions, patients often experience a long asymptomatic or 'latent' phase which may last decades. Assuming normal or supraphysiologic function, symptoms will vary with the regurgitant volume, which is determined by the ventricular–atrial pressure gradient (the driving pressure) and the size of the ERO. Not surprisingly, patients with moderate MR may notice only a slight limitation in ability to perform strenuous activities. With more advanced disease, net forward flow decreases while pulmonary venous pressure rises. This is manifest as fatigue and dyspnea with normal activities. With very advanced chronic MR, patients often develop palpitations (the result of atrial fibrillation) along with breathlessness and fatigue at rest (the result of severely elevated pulmonary venous pressure and diminished cardiac output).

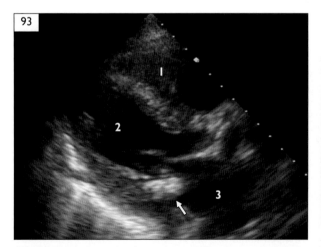
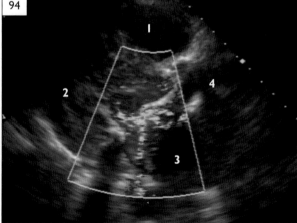

**93, 94** Posterior mitral annular calcification associated with mitral regurgitation. **93** 2D parasternal long axis view. Note the thickened and densely echogenic character of the posterior annulus (arrow) with acoustic shadowing (black area) behind the annulus. **94** Doppler color imaging demonstrating a wide jet of regurgitant flow into the left atrium. 1: right ventricle; 2: left ventricle; 3: left atrium; 4: aortic root.

**95** Left ventricular diastolic pressure–volume relationships in volume overload. **A**: Classic rightward shift of compensated volume overload lesions; mitral, tricuspid, and aortic regurgitation being the most common (red line). With little change in wall thickness, the chamber is greatly enlarged, with myocardial cell slippage allowing a reduction in chamber stiffness and growth of the pericardium allowing increased intracavitary volumes to exist with a normal low pericardial pressure. **B**: Chamber stiffness increases when decompensation occurs in volume overload (red line). Often the myocardium has become myopathic and fibrotic. End-diastolic and end-systolic volume have risen. (Adapted from Braunwald E, Zipes DP, Libby P (eds) (2001). *Heart Disease*, 6th edn. p. 1656.)

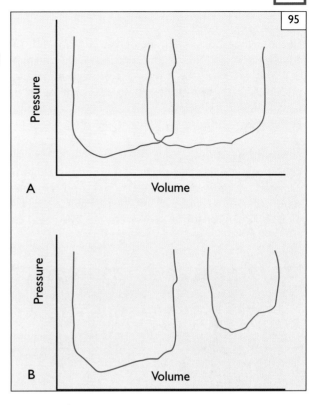

SIGNS

The physical findings will also vary with severity and chronicity of disease. Unless severely decompensated, the arterial pulses will be rapid in upstroke and blood pressure will be normal. Secondary pulmonary hypertension and right-sided failure will be manifest by elevated jugular venous pressure (JVP), peripheral edema, ascites, hepatic enlargement and congestion (positive hepatojugular reflux), and a sternal lift. In decompensated disease, crackles are typically found on lung auscultation and may be accompanied, inferiorly, by the percussed dullness of pleural effusions. As the LV dilates to accommodate the volume load, the apical impulse will be displaced laterally and is usually hyperkinetic. $S_1$ is often obscured by the MR murmur. $S_2$ may be paradoxically split due to a short LV ejection period. $P_2$ is often loud in pulmonary hypertension. An $S_3$ is commonly present and is best heard with the bell of the stethoscope with the patient in the left lateral decubitus position. The systolic murmur is classically holosystolic, but may be limited to late systole in mild functional MR. It is typically blowing in character, but can be harsh, is loudest at the apex, and radiates variably depending on the direction of the dominant regurgitant flow. In some cases, the murmur radiates to unusual locations including the back, neck, or skull. The regurgitant volume ($V_{regurg}$), added to the forward stroke volume, may comprise sufficient antegrade flow through the mitral valve to produce a low pitched diastolic rumble.

LABORATORY FINDINGS

*Electrocardiography*

The electrocardiogram (ECG) commonly includes findings of LA enlargement or atrial fibrillation. Left ventricular hypertrophy (LVH) and right ventricular hypertrophy (RVH) may also be apparent (**96**).

**96** 12-lead electrocardiogram demonstrating findings commonly seen in chronic mitral regurgitation: left atrial abnormality, left axis deviation, and left ventricular hypertrophy with repolarization abnormalities likely due to the ventricular hypertrophy. (Courtesy of Frances DeRook, MD.)

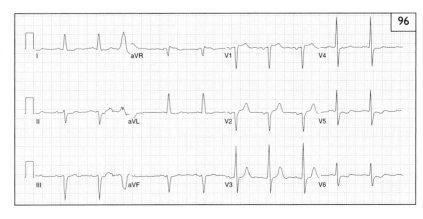

*Chest radiography*

Chest radiographs often demonstrate LA and LV enlargement (**97, 98**). Right ventricular enlargement may be seen in the presence of decompensated pulmonary hypertension. Left-sided heart failure is usually manifest by pulmonary vascular congestion and alveolar infiltrates.

*Echocardiography*

Echocardiography plays a central role in the evaluation of MR (Zoghbi *et al.*, 2003). 2D and Doppler echocardiography provide information regarding LA and LV, EF, mechanism and severity of MR, and by interrogating the velocity of the tricuspid regurgitation jet, an estimate of pulmonary artery systolic pressure (PASP) (**99–101**). Exercise echocardiography on a supine bicycle allows assessment of changes in MR and PASP during exercise. This can be particularly helpful in patients with severe exercise limitations, but near normal findings on resting echocardiography.

*Cardiac catheterization*

While echocardiography is the dominant diagnostic modality, cardiac catheterization and angiography (**102, 103**) can provide diagnostic information when clinical and echocardiographic data conflict. Though

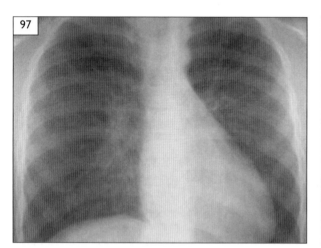

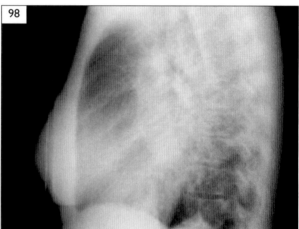

**97, 98** Postero-anterior and lateral chest films of a patient with combined mitral stenosis and mitral regurgitation. Left atrial enlargement is evidenced by the straightening of the left heart border (the loss of the normal concavity). (Courtesy of Bill Black, MD.)

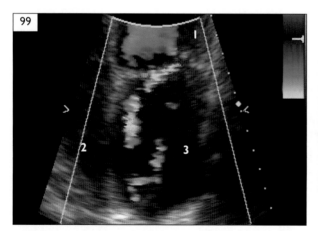

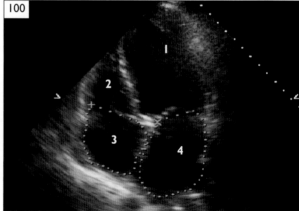

**99** Apical 4-chamber echocardiographic view showing a mitral regurgitant jet striking the interatrial septum. 1: left ventricle; 2: right atrium; 3: left atrium.

**100** Apical 4-chamber echocardiographic view demonstrating the left atrial enlargement (30.6 cm$^2$) which often accompanies chronic mitral regurgitation. 1: left ventricle; 2: right ventricle; 3: right atrium; 4: left atrium.

rarely performed in most laboratories, measurements can also be made during exercise as mentioned above. Catheterization is indicated prior to valve surgery in patients with atherosclerotic risk factors, to exclude the presence of coronary artery disease of sufficient severity to warrant surgical revascularization concomitant with the valve surgery.

The cardiac catheterization laboratory may also play an important therapeutic role in MR. By reducing ischemia, percutaneous coronary intervention (PCI) can dramatically impact on functional MR caused by arterial insufficiency. With the recent development of neointimal-inhibiting drug-eluting stents, it is expected that the role of PCI will continue to expand. In addition, percutaneously placed valves have already been used in humans in the aortic position (Cribier *et al*., 2003) and may someday have a role in mitral valve disease.

It is these data, combined with functional class, which guide decisions regarding mitral valve surgery.

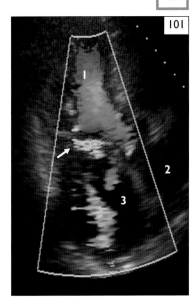

**101** Apical 3-chamber echocardiographic view showing a broad mitral regurgitant jet. 1: left ventricle; 2: aorta; 3: left atrium; arrow: mitral valve.

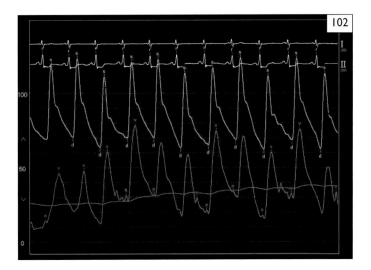

**102** Simultaneous pressure tracings from a pulmonary capillary wedge catheter and right femoral artery catheter. Note the large c-v wave.

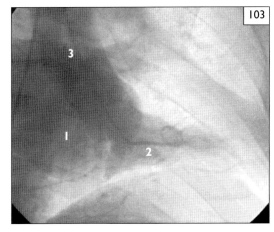

**103** Right anterior oblique projection of a left ventriculogram demonstrating opacification of the left atrium (1) following injection of contrast into the left ventricle (2) via a pigtail catheter placed retrograde via the ascending aorta (3).

## Medical management and follow-up

An algorithm for the management of chronic MR is shown in **104**. In brief, all patients with severe MR should be considered for surgical therapy with the exception of patients with severely decompensated LV failure (EF <30%) and asymptomatic patients with no sequelae (i.e. no atrial fibrillation; no pulmonary hypertension; an EF >60%; and an end-systolic diameter <45 mm) (Bonow *et al.*, 1998). Recommendations from a working group of the British Cardiac Society cite a slightly larger end-systolic criterion (55 mm) but suggest that earlier intervention may be favored when repair rather than replacement is being considered (Prendergast *et al.*, 1996). An alternative approach, consistent with previously cited European recommendations, is to use dimensions indexed to body surface area

(BSA) (Iung *et al.*, 2002). For chronic MR, an end-systolic dimension of 26 mm/m$^2$ has been suggested (Zile *et al.*, 1984).

Exercise should be limited to moderate levels in patients with symptoms or evidence of LV decompensation. Drug therapy serves little purpose in the management of this valve lesion. Since the LV is already 'unloaded' by the MR, vasodilating drugs such as angiotensin-converting enzyme (ACE) inhibitors or angiotensin receptor blockers (ARBs) would not be expected to improve prognosis or to reduce symptoms. The exception is MR caused by the geometric distortion produced by ischemic or dilated cardiomyopathy and in those cases where MR is exacerbated by hypertension. Atrial fibrillation should be managed with rate control and anticoagulation (Blackshear *et al.*, 1993). European guidelines differ

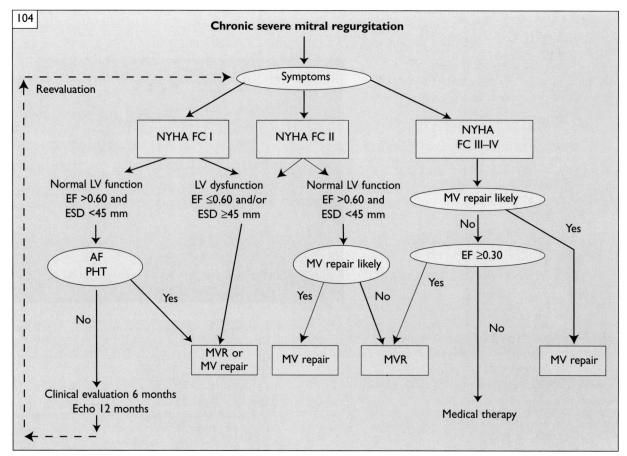

**104** Management strategy for patients with chronic severe mitral regurgitation. AF: atrial fibrillation; EF: ejection fraction; ESD: end-systolic diameter; FC: functional class; LV: left ventricle; MV: mitral valve; MVR: mitral valve replacement; NYHA: New York Heart Association; PHT: pulmonary hypertension. (Adapted from Bonow RO, Carabello B, de Leon AC Jr, *et al.* (1998). ACC/AHA guidelines for the management of patients with valvular heart disease. *Journal of the American College of Cardiology* 32:1486–1588.)

slightly from US guidelines by their slightly higher anticoagulation target (international normalized ratio [INR] 2.5–3.5) (Gohlke-Bärwolf *et al.*, 1995).

Symptomatic patients with moderate MR should be seen every 12 months and have echocardiograms every 24 months, while those asymptomatic patients with severe MR but no indication for surgery should be seen every 6 months, with echocardiograms every 12 months. Very close follow-up (every 6 months) is also recommended

for those patients approaching the accepted end-systolic and EF thresholds for surgery (Iung *et al.*, 2002). Patients should also be instructed to contact their physicians if they develop symptoms.

**Surgical intervention**

Three general types of operation exist: (i) mitral valve repair (**105**); (ii) mitral valve replacement (MVR) with tissue or mechanical valve prosthesis and preservation of the subvalvular apparatus (**106**); and (iii) MVR with excision of the subvalvular apparatus. In nonischemic MR, mitral valve repair is preferred as it avoids the possibility of tissue valve degeneration and thromboembolism associated with mechanical valves. In addition, it appears to be associated with lower perioperative mortality, improved survival, and better postoperative LV

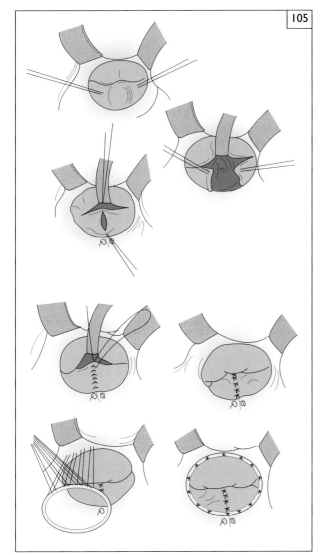

**105** Valve repair techniqes for quadrilateral resection of the posterior leaflet of the mitral valve. (Adapted from Cohn LH, DiSesa VJ, Couper GS, *et al.* (1989). Mitral valve repair for myxomatous degeneration and prolapse of the mitral valve. *Journal of Thoracic and Cardiovascular Surgery* **98**:987–993.)

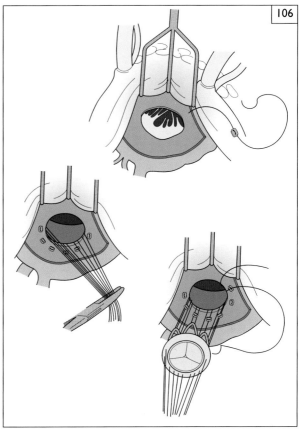

**106** Mitral valve replacement with preservation of the posterior leaflet. This preserves the annular-apical connection by means of the chordae tendineae. (Adapted from Albertucci M, Karp RB (1994). Prosthetic valve replacement. In: *Valvular Heart Disease*. M Al Zaibag, CMG Duran (eds). Marcel Dekker, New York, p. 613.)

function (Lee *et al.*, 1997). However, it may not always be possible to perform repair in rheumatic and ischemic valve disease or in the presence of significant calcification. Posterior leaflet prolapse and chordal rupture are usually amenable to repair (Gillinov and Cosgrove, 2002). Surgery is justified, in part, on the basis of data suggesting no excess mortality in patients undergoing valve surgery while in functional classes I–II (Tribouilloy *et al.*, 1999).

In ischemic MR, replacement may be superior to repair (DeAnda *et al.*, 2003). If MVR is performed, every effort should be made to preserve the subvalvular mitral apparatus as this technique appears to provide better postoperative LV function (Reardon and David, 1999) (**107**).

Technical success in well-selected patients may lead to dramatic improvement in LV dilatation (**108, 109**). Continued follow-up is indicated to monitor for valve repair failure (early), tissue valve deterioration (late), adequacy of anticoagulation in mechanical prosthesis (indefinite), and the development of atrial fibrillation or LV dysfunction (anytime).

## Case study

A 77-year-old male retired real estate agent saw a young internist to establish medical care following the sudden death of his previous physician. The patient had had a number of difficulties since retirement, starting with an inferior ST elevation myocardial infarction 5 years earlier. Despite prompt primary angioplasty of an occluded posterior descending artery, he was left with a dense inferior wall motion abnormality and an ejection fraction of 50%. He was treated with a beta-blocker for 1 year, a diuretic, digoxin, and aspirin. One year later he had a transient ischemic attack which led to the discovery of critical carotid stenosis and subsequent carotid artery stenting. Two years later he was found to have blood is his stool and a Duke stage B colon cancer was resected.

On this first visit with his new physician, the patient mentioned that he was having moderate shortness of breath climbing the stairs from his basement. He felt he had less energy than he had 1 year previously. Occasionally, he had some lightheadedness and ankle edema.

On exam, he was a very pleasant man who appeared younger than his stated age with a regular pulse of 89 bpm and a blood pressure of 166/84 mmHg (22.1/11.2 kPa). His estimated right atrial pressure was 12 cm of $H_2O$ with a prominent a wave. Crackles at his lung bases cleared with coughing.

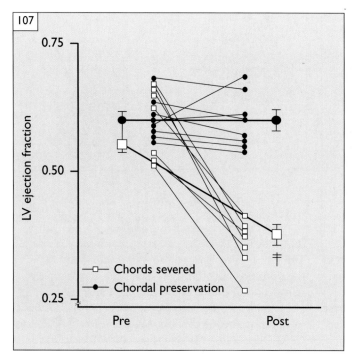

**107** Preoperative (Pre) and postoperative (Post) left ventricular (LV) ejection fractions for patients undergoing mitral valve replacement with chordae tendineae severed (open squares) or with chordae tendineae preserved (closed circles). (Adapted from Rozich JD, Carabello BA, Usher BW, *et al.* (1992). Mitral valve replacement with and without chordal preservation in patients with chronic mitral regurgitation: mechanisms for differences in postoperative ejection performance. *Circulation* **86**:1718–1726.)

There was no RV lift. His point of maximal intensity (PMI) was not displaced. $S_1$ was soft and $P_2$ was loud. He had a soft $S_4$ but no $S_3$. There was a 2/6 holosystolic murmur at the apex, radiating to the axilla. A well-healed midline abdominal incision was noted but he had no intra-abdominal masses or organomegaly. His complete blood count and serum chemistries including renal, liver, and thyroid function tests were all normal. He was started on carvedilol, lisinopril, and atorvastatin. His digoxin and furosemide were continued.

Two years later he was admitted to the hospital with left arm and wrist pain accompanied by dyspnea and diaphoresis. His ECG showed anterolateral ST depression and his troponins, but not his creatinine kinase levels, were elevated. He was treated with antiplatelet and antithrombin agents and brought to the catheterization lab where a 90% left main stenosis was found. There was moderately severe instent restenosis of the bare metal stent in the right coronary. An echocardiogram revealed mild anterolateral hypokinesis, inferior wall akinesis, an estimated ejection fraction of 45% with moderate left atrial enlargement, moderate left ventricular dilatation, and moderate-severe MR characterized by a vena contracta of 0.5 cm, blunting of pulmonary vein flow in systole, an early diastolic filling wave of 1.5 m/s, and an estimated left ventricular inflow stroke volume 50% greater than left ventricular outflow tract stroke volume. Mitral valve morphology appeared normal. The regurgitation was attributed to leaflet tethering and annular dilatation.

The next day he was taken for surgery and underwent two vessel bypass (left internal thoracic to left anterior descending and right internal thoracic to right posterior descending artery) and a mitral annuloplasty with a flexible ring. Save some postoperative atrial fibrillation, his subsequent course was uncomplicated. He played golf with his cardiothoracic intensive care nurse 3 months later.

COMMENTS

In this vignette, the origin, course, and definitive treatment of chronic MR due to ischemic heart disease is presented. Since it has a single vessel blood supply, the posteromedial papillary muscle is more suspectible to ischemic-/infarction-related dysfunction. This patient functioned well despite probable moderate MR following his first myocardial infarction, but his subsequent ischemic event lead to decompensation. His need for revascularization provided a excellent opportunity for annuloplasty. Despite the finding of carotid stenosis, one has to wonder if his transient ischemic attack was related to occult paroxysmal atrial fibrillation.

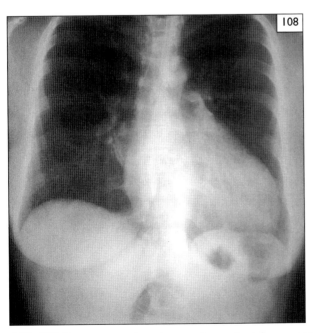 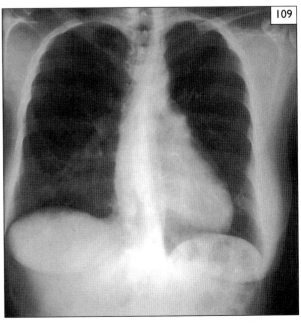

**108, 109** Postero-anterior chest radiographs taken preoperatively (**108**) and 6 weeks postoperatively (**109**) following mitral valve repair, demonstrating a dramatic reduction in cardiomegaly. (Courtesy of John Sanders, MD.)

## References

Blackshear JL, Pearce LA, Asinger RW, *et al.* (1993). Mitral regurgitation associated with reduced thromboembolic events in high-risk patients with nonrheumatic atrial fibrillation: Stroke Prevention in Atrial Fibrillation Investigators. *American Journal of Cardiology* 72:840–843.

Bonow RO, Carabello B, de Leon AC Jr, *et al.* (1998). ACC/AHA guidelines for the management of patients with valvular heart disease: a report of the American College of Cardiology/American Heart Association Task Force on Practice Guidelines (Committee on Management of Patients with Valvular Heart Disease). *Journal of the American College of Cardiology* 32:1486–1588.

Cribier A, Eltchaninoff H, Tron C (2003). [First human transcatheter implantation of an aortic valve prosthesis in a case of severe calcific aortic stenosis]. *Annales de Cardiologie et d'Angeiologie* 52(3):173–175.

DeAnda A Jr, Kasirajan V, Higgins RS (2003). Mitral valve replacement versus repair in 2003: where do we stand? *Current Opinion in Cardiology* 18(2):102–105.

Gillinov AM, Cosgrove DM (2002). Mitral valve repair for degenerative disease. *Journal of Heart Valve Disease* 11(Supplement 1):S15–20.

Gohlke-Bärwolf C, Acar J, Oakley C, *et al.* (1995). Guidelines for prevention of thromboembolic events in valvular heart disease. Study group of the Working Group on valvular heart disease of the European Society of Cardiology. *European Heart Journal* 16:1320–1330.

Grigioni F, Enriquez-Sarano M, Ling L, *et al.* (1999). Sudden cardiac death in mitral regurgitation due to flail leaflet. *Journal of the American College of Cardiology* 34:2078–2085.

Grossman W, Jones D, McLaurin LP (1975). Wall stress and patterns of hypertrophy in the human left ventricle. *Journal of Clinical Investigation* 56:56–64.

Iung B, Gohlke-Bärwolf C, Tornos P, *et al.* on behalf of the Working Group on Valvular Heart Disease (2002). Recommendations on the management of the asymptomatic patient with valvular heart disease. *European Heart Journal* 23(16):1253–1266.

Koelling TM, Aaronson KD, Cody RJ, Bach DS, Armstrong WF (2002). Prognostic significance of mitral regurgitation and tricuspid regurgitation in patients with left ventricular systolic function. *American Heart Journal* 144(3):524–529.

Lee EM, Shapiro LM, Wells FC (1997). Superiority of mitral valve repair in surgery for degenerative mitral regurgitation. *European Heart Journal* 18:655–663.

Ling H, Enriquez-Sarano M, Seward J, *et al.* (1996). Clinical outcomes of mitral regurgitation due to flail leaflets. *New England Journal of Medicine* 335:1417–1423.

Prendergast B, Banning AP, Hall RJC (1996). Valvular heart disease: recommendations for investigation and management. Summary of guidelines produced by a working group of the British Cardiac Society and the Research Unit of the Royal College of Physicians. *Journal of the Royal College of Physicians of London* 30:309–315.

Reardon MJ, David TE (1999). Mitral valve replacement with preservation of the subvalvular apparatus. *Current Opinion in Cardiology* 14(2):104–110.

Tribouilloy CM, Enriquez-Sarano M, Schaff HV, *et al.* (1999). Impact of preoperative symptoms on survival after surgical correction of organic mitral regurgitation: rationale for optimizing surgical indications. *Circulation* 99:400–405.

Tribouilloy CM, Enriquez-Sarano M, Capps MA, Bailey KR, Tajik AJ (2002).Contrasting effect of similar effective regurgitant orifice area in mitral and tricuspid regurgitation: a quantitative Doppler echocardiographic study. *Journal of the American Society of Echocardiography* 15(9):958–965.

Trichon BH, O'Connor CM (2002). Secondary mitral and tricuspid regurgitation accompanying left ventricular systolic dysfunction: is it important, and how is it treated? (editorial) *American Heart Journal* 144(3):373–376.

Zile MR, Gaasch WH, Carroll JD, Chan MR (1984). Predictive value of preoperative echocardiographic indexes of left ventricular function and wall stress. *Journal of the American College of Cardiology* 3:235–242.

Zoghbi WA, Enriquez-Sarano M, Foster E, *et al.* (2003). American Society of Echocardiography. Recommendations for evaluation of the severity of native valvular regurgitation with two-dimensional and Doppler echocardiography. *Journal of the American Society of Echocardiography* 16(7):777–802.

# Chapter Ten

# Acute Mitral Regurgitation

## Definition

Acute mitral regurgitation (MR) refers to retrograde flow through the mitral valve (MV) during ventricular systole, present for hours to weeks. Severity is measured as described in the previous chapter on chronic MR.

## Etiology

Not surprisingly, the causes of acute MR are usually themselves acute illnesses and can be placed into three broad categories: (i) inflammatory or rheumatologic diseases; (ii) infectious diseases; and (iii) ischemic syndromes. The rheumatologic causes of acute valve dysfunction include the inflammatory forms of arthritis, systemic lupus erythematosus, vasculitic syndromes (e.g. Kawasaki's disease and polyarteritis nodosa), and rheumatic fever (Bloom and Smith, 2002). Unusually, acute MR results from the sudden rupture of abnormal connective tissue in conditions which include Ehlers–Danlos, pseudoxanthum elasticum, Marfan syndrome, osteogenesis imperfecta, and Hurlers syndrome (110). Infectious causes of acute MR include bacterial and fungal endocarditis of both native and prosthetic valves. The mechanisms may include perforation of valve leaflets, perivalvular leaks, failure to coapt due to bulky vegetations, and unseating of the valve. The ischemic etiologies include MR due to severe wall motion abnormalities and MR due to infarction of papillary muscles or chords. Most often, the ischemia is the result of atherosclerotic

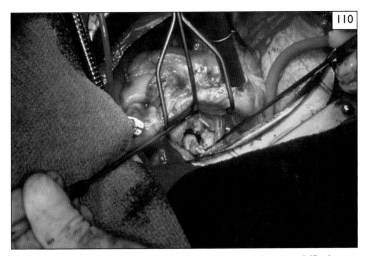

**110** Intraoperative photograph of a patient with acute MR due to ruptured chordae tendineae. Note the strands of free chordae. (Courtesy of John Sanders, MD.)

coronary artery disease. However, it is important to recognize that there are other causes of ischemia such as vasculitis or thrombophilia (111–115). Failure of a bioprosthetic valve is another cause of acute MR.

Frequently, a distinction is made between *organic* and *functional* MR. In the former, there is an anatomic abnormality of the valve itself, whereas in the latter, valve leak occurs as a result of abnormalities in the supporting apparatus.

### Pathophysiology

Incomplete coaptation of the mitral valve creates a regurgitant orifice. The volume of retrograde flow through this orifice is known as the regurgitant volume. Dividing this volume by the total amount ejected by the left ventricle (LV) yields the regurgitant fraction (Rahimtoola *et al.*, 2001).

In acute MR, this regurgitant fraction is ejected into a noncompliant left atrium (LA). As a result, the regurgitant volume produces a sharp increase in LA pressure manifest on a Swan Ganz tracing as a V wave. This pressure is transmitted to the pulmonary venous system resulting in vascular congestion, interstitial edema and, if sufficiently high, alveolar edema. Accompanying this increase in atrial pressure is an increase in natriuretic peptides and activation of the renin–angiotensin system.

Different burdens are placed on the ventricle and the systemic arterial circulation. Like acute aortic regurgitation (AR) (see Chapter 6), a sudden volume burden is placed on the LV. However, because regurgi-

tant flow occurs during systole, it is of shorter duration; since the v wave limits the pressure differential between the ventricle and the atrium, the rate of regurgitant flow tends to be less than in acute AR. These two factors generally explain the smaller regurgitant volume per regurgitant orifice area in acute MR as compared to acute AR (Rahimtoola *et al.*, 2001).

With stroke volume preferentially ejected into the LA, forward flow drops, resulting in an accompanying sudden decrease in systemic cardiac output and tissue perfusion.

### Clinical presentation
#### SYMPTOMS

Symptoms vary with the size of the regurgitant volume. Mild MR (regurgitant volume <20 ml) is usually well tolerated even if it develops suddenly. A limitation in ability to perform strenuous tasks may be all that is noticed. Moderate MR (regurgitant volume 20–40 ml) commonly produces fatigue and dyspnea with normal activities. Atrial fibrillation, precipitated by stretch of the LA, may produce palpitations. At the extreme end of acute MR (volume >60 ml) typified by rupture of a papillary muscle (116), patients often present with the sudden onset of atypical chest pain, cardiogenic shock, and pulmonary edema. In acute MR due to a reversible cause (e.g. ischemic papillary dysfunction), a patient may present with pulmonary edema which clears rapidly with diuresis and antianginal therapy.

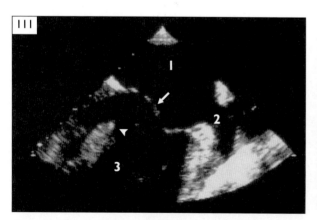 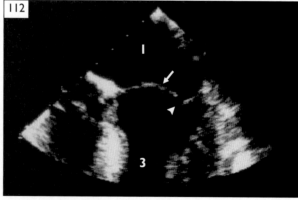

**111, 112** Transesophageal echocardiography. **111** Posterior displacement of the anterior mitral valve leaflet (arrow) and failure of coaptation of the anterior and posterior leaflets (arrowhead). The papillary muscle is echodense and elongated. **112** View (rotated 90° from the view in **111**) shows that the posteromedial papillary muscle (arrowhead) is elongated and that there is prolapse of the anterior mitral valve leaflet (arrow). 1: left atrium; 2: left atrial appendage; 3: left ventricle. (Reprinted from Bloom BJ, Smith RN (2002). Weekly clinicopathological exercises: case 29-2002: a 17-year-old boy with acute mitral regurgitation and pulmonary edema. *New England Journal of Medicine* **347**(12):921–928. With permission. Copyright Massachusetts Medical Society. All rights reserved.)

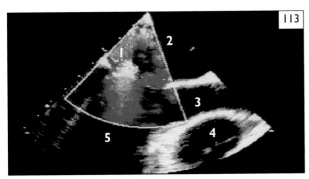

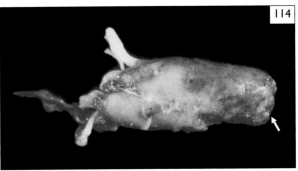

**113** Doppler color flow transesophageal echocardiography. Severe, posteriorly directed mitral regurgitation (1) is visible as a band of orange flecked with yellow. 2: left atrium; 3: left ventricular outflow; 4: right ventricular outflow; 5: left ventricle. (Reprinted from Bloom BJ, Smith RN (2002). Weekly clinicopathological exercises: case 29-2002: a 17-year-old boy with acute mitral regurgitation and pulmonary edema. *New England Journal of Medicine* **347**(12):921–928. With permission. Copyright Massachusetts Medical Society. All rights reserved.)

**114** Ruptured papillary muscle. The arrow shows the rupture site. The chordae are on the left-hand side of the specimen. The muscle is pale yellow and soft, with some focal hyperemia. The gross findings are consistent with the development of an infarct 3–5 days before the rupture. (Reprinted from Bloom BJ, Smith RN (2002). Weekly clinicopathological exercises: case 29-2002: a 17-year-old boy with acute mitral regurgitation and pulmonary edema. *New England Journal of Medicine* **347**(12):921–928. With permission. Copyright Massachusetts Medical Society. All rights reserved.)

**115** Necrotic myocardium (upper left), with loss of nuclei (hematoxylin and eosin, ×200). Infiltrating neutrophils are present at the border of the infarct. The inset (hematoxylin and eosin, ×1000) shows contraction band necrosis. These microscopic findings are consistent with the development of an infarct 3–5 days before the rupture. (Reprinted from Bloom BJ, Smith RN (2002). Weekly clinicopathological exercises: case 29-2002: a 17-year-old boy with acute mitral regurgitation and pulmonary edema. *New England Journal of Medicine* **347**(12):921–928. With permission. Copyright Massachusetts Medical Society. All rights reserved.)

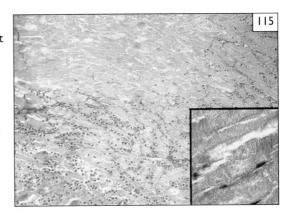

**116** Papillary muscle rupture. Transesophageal view of a flail anterior mitral leaflet resulting from rupture of a papillary muscle. A portion of the papillary muscle is seen whipping into the left atrium still attached to the chordae tendineae of this leaflet (arrow). The sudden onset of the associated mitral regurgitation generally causes pulmonary edema and necessitates emergent surgery. 1: left atrium; 2: left ventricle.

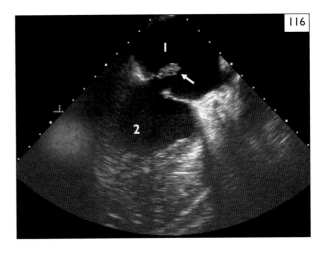

SIGNS

As with symptoms, the physical exam varies with the severity of the MR. In severe acute MR, patients typically present with a general appearance of distress and apprehension, a very upright posture, cool and diaphoretic skin, and moderate respiratory distress. In less severe cases, these findings will be absent. Blood pressure is usually normal and the carotid upstroke is brisk.

The apical impulse is hyperdynamic but, without time for LV dilatation, it will not be displaced. Large volume MR may produce a thrill palpable over the apex. If sufficient to produce acute pulmonary hypertension, right ventricular (RV) dilatation may develop and be manifest as a sternal lift. $S_1$ is usually subsumed with the MR murmur. $S_2$ may be persistently split if LV ejection time is particularly short. By adding to the antegrade flow through the MV, the regurgitant volume contributes to rapid and high volume filling of the LV. This can sometimes be detected as an $S_3$ and a diastolic flow rumble. The systolic murmur of MR is usually holosystolic, though in cases of mild functional MR the mitral leaflets may only fail to coapt at higher ventricular volumes. For this reason, the murmur may be limited to early systole in mild functional MR. The murmur is usually blowing, but this is somewhat variable, and it may be harsh. It is usually loudest at the apex. The direction of radiation will depend on the direction of the regurgitant jet. For example, prolapse of the anterior leaflet will direct the flow posteriorly, hence producing a murmur which radiates to the axilla. Conversely, prolapse of the posterior leaflet will direct flow anteriorly and medially, producing a murmur which radiates to the base of the heart. In some cases, a murmur of MR radiates to the back, neck, or skull based upon the direction of regurgitant flow.

LABORATORY FINDINGS

Upon completion of physical examination, patients with severe acute MR in heart failure should be further assessed by urgent laboratory studies including arterial blood gas analysis, chest radiography, electrocardiography (ECG), and transthoracic echocardiography. If there is any doubt about the severity or mechanism of the MR by transthoracic echo, transesophageal echocardiography (TEE) should be considered.

As in chronic MR, echocardiography is the mainstay of both qualitative and quantitative assessment. Organic and functional MR can be distinguished by using 2D imaging to assess valve morphology. Color flow Doppler imaging can provide semiquantitative assessment of the degree of MR, based on the percent of LA area penetrated by regurgitant flow. More strictly quantitative methods of assessing MR are based on intracardiac volumetric flow, but these are beyond the scope of this handbook. Although infrequently used, radionuclide studies can be used to estimate the stroke volumes of both ventricles and, by subtraction, provide the regurgitant volume.

With the growing sophistication of echocardiographic methods, the catheterization laboratory is increasingly reserved for preoperative assessment of obstructive coronary disease. However, the hemodynamic consequences of MR can be documented precisely and semiquantitative techniques can be employed to grade the degree of MR.

## Medical management

If the MR is severe, the management is primarily surgical. If the patient's general medical condition does not preclude surgery, no time should be lost seeking cardiothoracic surgical consultation. While awaiting surgery, medical management includes obtaining preoperative laboratory work, maintenance of oxygenation with intubation and mechanical ventilation as needed, and encouraging forward flow by reducing afterload pharmacologically with vasodilators, or mechanically with an intra-aortic balloon pump (**117–119**).

In more mild cases of acute MR, treatment with diuretics and vasodilators as well as prompt management of atrial fibrillation may provide time for the LA to stretch and become more compliant, hence allowing the patient to reach a stage of compensated chronic MR. These patients will require ongoing surveillance to treat any complications (e.g. atrial fibrillation) promptly and to identify possible indications for surgery.

## Surgical intervention

The surgical options in treating MR are outlined in Chapter 9 and include MV repair or replacement (MVR). As in chronic MR, valve repair is preferred when it is technically feasible. Surgical exposure can be achieved by a traditional median sternotomy or by a newer 'minimally-invasive' approach. If MVR is selected, the decision to implant a tissue or a mechanical prosthesis will be contingent principally upon the patient's life expectancy and any pre-existing need for anticoagulation.

## Case study

A 33-year-old former gymnast suddenly became dyspneic and overcome with a sense of doom while

**117–119** Intra-aortic balloon pump. **117** The device is inserted in the femoral artery and positioned in the descending thoracic aorta. By rapidly deflating during systole and inflating during diastole, it reduces afterload and augments diastolic pressure. **118** Control console for the intra-aortic balloon pump. **119** Display of electrocardiogram and pressure tracing from the intra-aortic balloon pump. The top tracing is a single lead rhythm strip demonstrating atrial fibrillation. The second line is a display of intra-aortic pressure with 1:1 native beat to balloon inflations. The smaller peak immediately following the R wave is the pressure rise generated by ventricular systole. The taller second peak is created by the balloon inflating during diastole. The bottom tracing represents balloon inflation pressure with time. (Photos courtesy of Toray Industries Inc.)

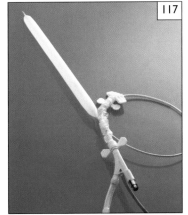

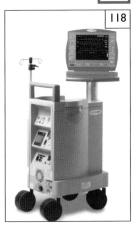

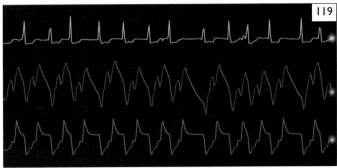

helping a friend lift a table saw into the back of a pickup truck. She developed increasing respiratory distress and lost consciousness over the subsequent 10 minutes; she was breathing but not responsive. The emergency medical service was activated and arrived at the remote construction site within 20 minutes. She was intubated and normal saline was administered via two large bore intravenous lines. Upon arrival in the local emergency room she was mottled and remained unresponsive. Pink frothy sputum was suctioned frequently from her endotracheal tube. Her pulse was 145 bpm and regular. Systolic blood pressure was 60 mmHg (8 kPa). Her lung exam revealed diffuse crackles. Her neck veins were distended. Her heart sounds were very tachycardic with no discernible murmur. An ECG demonstrated a sinus tachycardia without ST elevation. Initial blood counts were normal.

No emergent echocardiographic or catheterization facilities existed at this rural hospital. Air transport to a tertiary center was requested but was not available because of fog. The local physician accompanied her in the ambulance to the nearest medical center. Two minutes into the trip the patient's blood pressure dropped below a level detectable by stethoscope. Her monitor showed atrial fibrillation with rapid ventricular reponse. Despite additional fluids, DC cardioversion,

epinephrine (adrenaline), dopamine, and amiodarone for subsequent ventricular tachycardia and fibrillation, 60 minutes of resuscitation efforts in the ambulance and the receiving hospital emergency room were unsuccessful.

A postmortem examination revealed a ruptured primary chorde tendinae and pulmonary edema. A generalized disorder of connective tissue was diagnosed as probable Ehlers–Danlos syndrome.

COMMENTS

This tragic case exemplifies the potentially catastrophic nature of acute severe MR. The remote location of this woman's collapse and the lack of facilities to insert an intra-aortic balloon pump greatly disadvantaged her prognosis.

**References**

Bloom BJ, Smith RN (2002). Weekly clinicopathological exercises: case 29-2002: a 17-year-old boy with acute mitral regurgitation and pulmonary edema. *New England Journal of Medicine* 347(12):921–928.

Rahimtoola SH, Enriquez-Sarano M, Schaff HV, *et al.* (2001). Mitral valve disease. In: *Hurst's The Heart*, 10th edn. V Fuster, RW Alexander, RA O'Rourke, *et al.* (eds). McGraw-Hill, New York, pp. 1697–1728.

# Chapter Eleven

# Pulmonic Stenosis

## Definition

As with the aortic valve, pulmonic stenosis (PS) may be considered more broadly as right ventricular (RV) outflow track obstruction with supravalvular, valvular, and subvalvular forms. It is commonly graded on the basis of peak pressure gradient: (i) trivial (<25 mmHg, 3.3 kPa); (ii) mild (25–49 mmHg, 3.3–6.5 kPa); (iii) moderate (50–79 mmHg, 6.7 kPa); and (iv) severe (≥80 mmHg, 10.7 kPa).

## Etiology

The most common causes of PS are related to congenital anomalies of the valve. While valvular PS often occurs in isolation, supra- and subvalvular stenosis usually comprise part of a larger syndrome (Therrien and Webb, 2001) (**120, 121**). Acquired causes of PS include rheumatic heart disease (very rare), carcinoid syndrome, and extrinsic compression from tumors (**122, 123**) or aneurysms

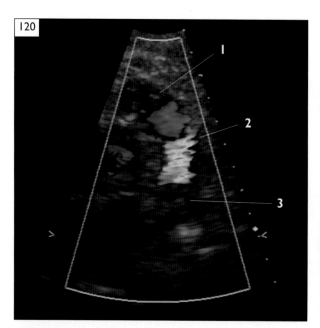

**120** Doppler color flow imaging from a parasternal short axis echocardiographic perspective, demonstrating high velocity flow in the main pulmonary artery in supravalvular pulmonic stenosis. 1: right ventricular outflow tract; 2: high velocity supravalvular jet; 3: main pulmonary artery.

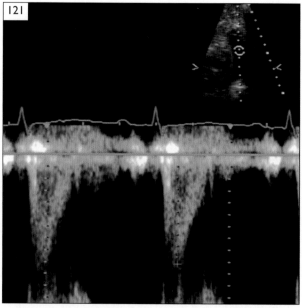

**121** Pulse wave Doppler in the pulmonary artery demonstrating a velocity of 1.8 m/sec in supravalvular pulmonic stenosis.

of the sinuses of Valsalva. Other rare causes include myocardial sarcomas and myxomas, and scarring following previous pulmonary valve surgery. Isolated peripheral pulmonary artery stenosis can mimic valvular PS.

### Pathophysiology

Pulmonary stenosis places a pressure load on the RV, which elicits concentric hypertrophy. This increase in wall thickness serves to moderate increases in wall tension produced by elevated intracavitary pressure (Laplace's law: wall tension = [pressure × radius]/ 2 × wall thickness). As in aortic stenosis (AS), the concentric hypertrophy is accompanied by an increase in collagen and impaired diastolic function. Consequently, RV end-diastolic pressure (RVEDP) begins to rise while systolic function remains normal. This is transmitted to the right atrium (RA) and systemic veins. In the face of longstanding or progressive PS, systolic RV dysfunction develops. Due, in part, to the crescentic geometry of the RV, this develops at lower levels of valve resistance than seen in the left ventricle (LV). As in other causes of

right heart failure, RA pressure increases are transmitted to the systemic venous system and cause passive congestion of the liver, gut, spleen, and dependent extremities.

While trivial amounts of tricuspid regurgitation (TR) are detected in most healthy individuals, it becomes increasingly severe in the presence of rising RV pressure. Employing the simplified Bernoulli equation (pressure = 4 × velocity$^2$), the velocity of this regurgitant flow as measured by Doppler echocardiography can be used to estimate the pressure difference between the RV and the RA. By adding this pressure difference to an estimated or directly measured RA pressure, one can arrive at a reasonably accurate noninvasive estimate of RV pressure. Using this same equation, the pressure gradient across the stenotic valve may be estimated using the peak instantaneous velocity of blood flow across the stenotic valve.

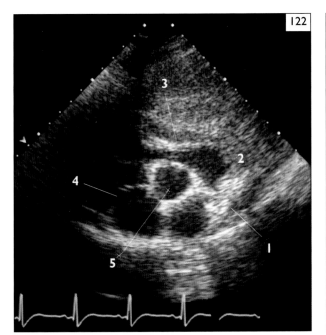 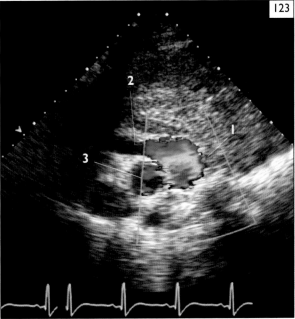

**122, 123** Supravalvular pulmonic stenosis due to extrinsic compression. **122** 2D parasternal short axis view at the base of the heart displaying extrinsic compression (1) of the pulmonary artery (2) distal to the valve (3). 4: tricuspid valve; 5: aortic valve. **123** Doppler color flow imaging from the same location as **122**, displaying acceleration of flow (1) proximal to the obstruction. 2: right ventricular outflow tract; 3: aortic valve.

## Clinical presentation

### SYMPTOMS

Mild PS is often asymptomatic. Patients with more severe stenosis commonly develop poor exercise tolerance, dyspnea, light-headedness, and may develop angina. Syncope is a rare and dramatic presentation of severe PS. Carcinoid valve disease is suggested by serotonin-mediated attacks of facial flushing, increased intestinal activity, wheezing, and diarrhea.

### SIGNS

On physical exam the decrease in RV compliance associated with RV hypertrophy (RVH) may be manifest as a prominent jugular a wave. RVH may produce a visible and palpable sternal lift. Turbulent flow across the stenotic valve produces a systolic ejection murmur loudest over the left second intercostal space, sometimes associated with a thrill. If the valve leaflets are pliable, an ejection click, diminished by inspiration, may be audible (Braunwald, 2001).

### LABORATORY FINDINGS

*Electrocardiography*

While not specific to PS, electrocardiographic (ECG) findings may include evidence of RVH (right axis deviation and an R wave greater than S wave in $V_1$) and right atrial enlargement (p wave amplitude >2.5 mm in lead II and >1.5 mm in $V_1$).

*Chest radiography*

Chest radiographs may reveal poststenotic dilatation of the main and left pulmonary arteries in valvular PS (**124, 125**).

*Echocardiography*

Echocardiography is the dominant technology used in the characterization of PS. 2D imaging by transthoracic or transesophageal approaches allows inspection of the valve morphology. Doppler color flow mapping and 2D-guided pulsed and continuous wave Doppler interrogation allow determination of the level of stenosis, the approximate peak pressure gradient (as described above), and the presence of any associated congenital anomalies.

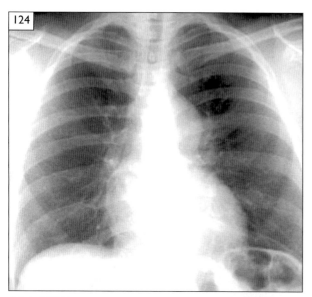

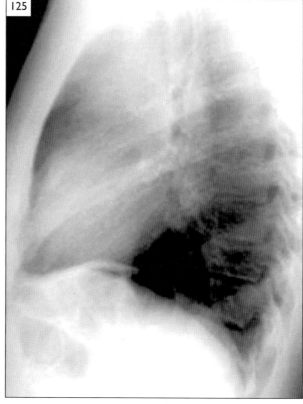

**124, 125** Postero-anterior (**124**) and lateral (**125**) chest films of a 29-year-old female with severe pulmonary stenosis (peak-to-peak pressure gradient by right heart catheterization of 70 mmHg [9.3 kPa]). Note the prominence of the main pulmonary artery resulting from poststenotic dilatation. (Courtesy of Bill Black, MD.)

## *Cardiac catheterization*

Cardiac catheterization provides confirmation of the pressure gradients (**126**), full hemodynamic assessment, and identification of associated pulmonary artery branch stenoses (Almeda *et al.*, 2003).

## Medical management

The usual considerations of endocarditis prophylaxis and rheumatic fever prophylaxis apply to PS. Right-sided heart failure can be treated with diuretics but therapy with these drugs should not be used to delay definitive treatment. As mentioned in other chapters, severe valvular disorders generally require mechanical solutions, hence surgical, not medical treatment, is appropriate. Atrial fibrillation should be promptly treated with atrioventricular node active agents (e.g. beta-blockers, non-dihydropyridine calcium channel blockers, digitalis) to achieve rate control, and warfarin to an international normalized ratio (INR) of 2–3 to prevent thromboembolic complications.

## Percutaneous and surgical intervention

Patients with severe PS were treated by surgical valvotomy until 1982, when percutaneous balloon valvuloplasty was developed (Kan *et al.*, 1982). This was a seminal development in the treatment of congenital heart disease and was relatively rapidly adopted by the pediatric community. However, its application in adolescents and adults took longer. The subsequent commercial availability of the two component, self-positioning Inoue balloon represented a further refinement of the technique. The efficacy of this technique was described in a review of 53 patients ranging from 13 to 55 years in age followed for an average of $7 \pm 3$ years (Chen *et al.*, 1996). Immediately after the procedure, the invasively measured systolic pressure gradient dropped from $91 \pm 46$ mmHg ($12.1 \pm 6.1$ kPa) to $38 \pm 32$ mmHg ($5.1 \pm 4.3$ kPa). The diameter of the valve orifice increased from $9 \pm 4$ mm to $17 \pm 5$ mm. By Doppler measurement, the systolic gradient decreased from $107 \pm 48$ mmHg ($14.3 \pm 6.4$ kPa) to $50 \pm 29$ mmHg ($6.7 \pm 3.9$ kPa) after valvuloplasty and at last follow-up remained at $30 \pm 16$ mmHg

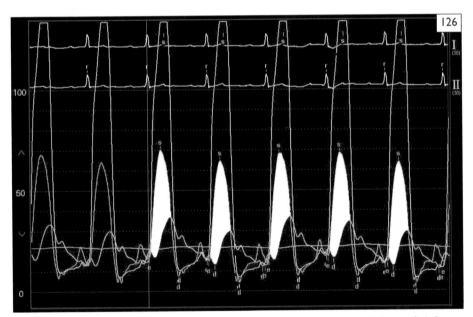

**126** Simultaneous invasive pressure tracings of the right ventricle (RV, green), left ventricle (yellow), and pulmonary artery (PA, blue) from a patient with severe pulmonary stenosis. Note the systolic pressure difference between the RV and PA represented by the shaded area.

(4 ± 2.1 kPa). Pulmonic valve incompetence was noted in 7 of 53 patients immediately after valvuloplasty, but was absent at follow-up exam in all patients.

Currently, balloon valvuloplasty is recommended for symptomatic patients and those with a peak gradient >50 mmHg (6.7 kPa). Surgical valvuloplasty is reserved for situations of severe valve calcification, severe dysplasia, previous repair of congenitally abnormal pulmonary valves, and uncontrolled endocarditis (Therrien and Webb, 2001). In instances of endocarditis and active illicit intravenous drug use, the optimal approach may be simple valvectomy.

### Case study

A 56-year-old electrician visited an urgent care center in a nearby retail 'super store' while buying some underwear, because he had developed frequent diarrheal stools. An antimotility agent was prescribed and he was counseled about possible aggravating dietary habits. Six months later he visited a family physician because of persistent diarrhea. Review of systems revealed that he also had episodic facial flushing and wheezing. An albuterol inhaler given to him by his brother had provided partial relief for the wheezing. He had no chronic health conditions other than psoriasis and obesity. He took no medications. None of his 1st degree relatives had any chronic gastrointestinal illnesses. Exam was remarkable only for a 4.5 kg (10 lb) weight loss. Stool studies, blood tests including a complete blood count, liver, renal, thyroid function tests, a test for celiac sprue, an upper gastrointestinal and small bowel follow-through contrast study, and sigmoidoscopy were performed. All studies, including sigmoid biopsy, came back normal.

Three months later, he returned with persistence of the above symptoms now accompanied by dyspnea on exertion, anorexia, increasing abdominal girth, and lower extremity edema. His weight was now up 6.75 kg (15 lb) from baseline. Pulse rate was 92 bpm and regular. Blood pressure was 115/66 mmHg (15.3/8.8 kPa) in both arms without pulsus paradoxus. His mean jugular venous pressure was estimated to be 10 cm above the sternal angle, with a prominent a wave. His chest was clear to percussion and auscultation. He had an RV lift with a thrill at the left upper sternal border. Auscultation revealed a soft $S_1$ at the left lower sternal border, a 2/6 holosystolic murmur at the left lower sternal border, and a 4/6 systolic ejection murmur loudest at the site of the thrill. He had an enlarged and subtly pulsatile liver, a fluid wave, and shifting dullness on percussion. Moderate pitting edema to midshin was noted.

Echocardiography revealed severe PS with estimated peak and mean pressure gradients of 74/35 mmHg (9.9/4.7 kPa), a dilated RV with global hypokinesis, and moderate tricuspid regurgitation. The pulmonic valve and tricuspid valves appeared fibrotic. Plaques were seen lining the RA and RV. The LV and the remaining valves were normal.

A 24-hour urine for 5-hydroxyindoleacetic acid was markedly elevated. Indium-111 octreotide scintigraphy revealed increased activity in the right lower quadrant. Computed tomography scan of the abdomen revealed multiple space-occupying lesions in the liver. The patient subsequently underwent percutaneous pulmonary balloon valvulotomy with immediate improvement in pressure gradients and decrease in tricuspid regurgitation. He then underwent laparotomy with resection of a 2 cm tumor from the appendix and debulking of his liver metastases.

### COMMENTS

This case illustrates the presentation, exam and laboratory findings, and course of a patient with right-sided valvular disease secondary to metastastic carcinoid tumor arising in the midgut. Unlike this case, TR usually dominates the clinical picture. Relief of RV outflow obstruction served to lessen somewhat the degree of TR. The prognosis in a case like this is guarded.

### References

Almeda FQ, Kavinsky CJ, Pophal SG, Klein LW (2003). Pulmonic valvular stenosis in adults: diagnosis and treatment. *Catheterization and Cardiovascular Interventions* 60(4):546–557.

Braunwald E (2001). Valvular heart disease. In: *Heart Disease: A Textbook of Cardiovascular Medicine*. E Braunwald, DP Zipes, P Libby (eds). WB Saunders, Philadelphia, ch 46, pp.1643–1722.

Chen C, Cheng T, Huang T, *et al.* (1996). Percutaneous balloon valvuloplasty for pulmonic stenosis in adolescents and adults. *New England Journal of Medicine* 335:21–25.

Kan JS, White RJ Jr, Mitchell SE, Gardner TJ (1982). Percutaneous balloon valvuloplasty: a new method for treating congenital pulmonary valve stenosis. *New England Journal of Medicine* 307:540–542.

Therrien J, Webb GD (2001). Congenital heart disease in adults. In: *Heart Disease: A Textbook of Cardiovascular Medicine*. E Braunwald, DP Zipes, P Libby (eds). WB Saunders, Philadelphia, ch 44, pp.1592–1621.

# Chapter Twelve

# Pulmonic Regurgitation

## Definition

Pulmonic regurgitation (PR) refers to retrograde flow across the pulmonic valve during diastole. Trivial amounts of PR are commonly observed in healthy adults and may be considered normal. Regurgitant flow in excess of this is graded on a 1–4 point scale. The grading system is discussed below in the sections addressing laboratory findings.

## Etiology

Analogous to aortic regurgitation, the most common cause of PR is dilatation of the pulmonary artery root, related to elevated pulmonary blood pressure. This may be secondary to any of the causes of pulmonary hypertension including left ventricular (LV) dysfunction, mitral valve (MV) disease, pulmonary venous occlusive disease, diffuse pulmonary parenchymal disease, chronic thrombo-embolic disease, and primary pulmonary hypertension. Alternatively, pulmonary root dilatation may arise from abnormal connective tissue in Ehlers–Danlos syndrome, pseudoxanthum elasticum, Marfan's syndrome, osteogenesis imperfecta, or Hurler's syndrome.

Congenital anomalies represent another broad category of causes. Complete absence of the pulmonary valve is rare and, when present, is often accompanied by a narrowed pulmonic annulus with rudimentary cusps, pulmonary artery dilatation, and a malaligned ventricular septal defect: a syndrome described as tetralogy of Fallot with absent pulmonary valve. Less commonly, absence of the pulmonary valve has been reported in conjunction with an atrial-septal defect (ASD), a patent ductus arteriosus, or both (Sayger et al., 2000). Very rarely, isolated congenital absence of the pulmonary valve is seen. Remarkably, it has been reported as an incidental finding on necropsy of a 73-year-old male who died as the result of a stroke (Pouget et al.,

1967). Still rarer is the isolated congenital absence of a single pulmonary valve cusp (Sayger et al., 2000). An echocardiogram from a patient with this anomaly is shown (127).

Other causes include infective endocarditis, syphilis, rheumatic heart disease, carcinoid, and trauma.

Whether pulmonary artery catheters cause or increase pulmonary artery regurgitation has been a source of debate in the past. However, this topic was recently studied (Sherman et al., 2001). In 54 anesthetized adult patients undergoing elective

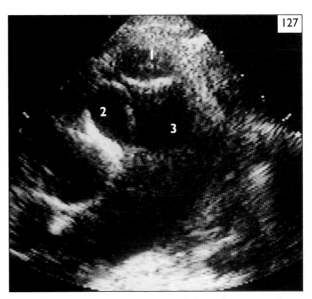

**127** Parasternal short-axis view of the pulmonary valve showing the absence of the left lateral facing leaflet.
1: right-facing leaflet; 2: anterior nonfacing leaflet; 3: absent left lateral-facing leaflet. (From Sayger P, Lewis M, Arcilla R, Ilbawi M (2000). Isolated congenital absence of a single pulmonary valve cusp. *Pediatric Cardiology* **21**:487–489. With permission of Springer Publishing.)

cardiovascular surgery, transesophageal echocardiography (TEE) was performed before and after passage of a pulmonary artery catheter. Patients with known PR or tricuspid regurgitation (TR) were excluded. Heart rate and blood pressure were not statistically different during the two assessments. The PR jet area was measured at the midesophageal. The mean increase in PR jet area was 0.12 cm$^2$ and was not statistically significant. Only 8% of patients had an increase in PR jet area >1 cm$^2$.

## Pathophysiology

In PR, the right heart is burdened with a volume load. To accommodate this increased volume, the right ventricle (RV) compensates by dilating. In the process, the tricuspid annulus may also become dilated. Both annular dilatation and remodeling of the RV (to which the tricuspid supporting apparatus is attached) inhibit the successful coaptation of the tricuspid valve leaflets, resulting in secondary TR. In this manner, PR begets TR.

If the underlying cause of the PR is pulmonary hypertension, the RV is subjected to a pressure load as well and compensatory adaptation may include increased wall thickness, which serves to diminish wall tension (Laplace's law: wall tension = [intracavitary pressure × radius]/× wall thickness). In pulmonary hypertension, the high pressure gradient between the RV and right atrium (RA) results in high velocity TR flow (modified Bernoulli equation: pressure = 4V$^2$). Large volume TR may lead to RA dilatation and a predisposition to atrial fibrillation.

## Clinical presentation

### SYMPTOMS

Symptoms generally reflect the proximate disease (e.g. pulmonary hypertension, infective endocarditis) rather than the PR itself. However, if decompensated, patients may develop symptoms of right heart failure including easy fatiguability, dyspnea on exertion (from diminished cardiac output), weight gain, and peripheral edema (from elevated systemic venous pressure), right upper quadrant discomfort (from hepatic congestion and stretch of the hepatic capsule), as well as nausea, vomiting, anorexia, and abdominal bloating (from portal venous hypertension).

### SIGNS

Physical findings will vary with the severity of PR. General physical findings may include peripheral edema, ascites, hepatomegaly, and elevated jugular venous pressure with a prominent c-v wave. The RV may produce a sternal lift and the increased RV stroke

volume may produce exaggerated pulmonary artery (PA) distension, palpable in the left second intercostal space. In pulmonary hypertension, the prolonged RV ejection period may produce a widely split S$_2$ with a loud pulmonary component (P$_2$). A systolic ejection click may be heard in the presence of a dilated PA. In advanced disease, RV dilatation and decreased compliance may produce right-sided third and fourth heart sounds. With normal pulmonary artery pressures, a brief, low-pitched, diastolic murmur, louder with inspiration, is heard in the left third and fourth intercostal spaces. With pulmonary hypertension, a Graham–Steell murmur may be audible as an early diastolic, high-pitched, blowing, decrescendo murmur along the left parasternal border (128). Differentiation from aortic regurgitation (AR) is aided by the absence of a widened pulse pressure (Braunwald, 2001).

### LABORATORY FINDINGS

#### Electrocardiography

Electrocardiography (ECG) may reveal an rSr pattern in V$_1$ (suggestive of RV diastolic overload) and possible right axis deviation. Pulmonary hypertension may produce ECG evidence of right ventricular hypertrophy (129).

#### Chest radiography

Chest films often show evidence of RV dilatation, which is best seen on the lateral view as loss of the retrosternal 'clear space'. As noted above, the PA may be dilated.

#### Echocardiography

2D and Doppler echocardiography, supplemented as needed by transesophageal imaging, can provide information about valve morphology, associated congenital anomalies, chamber size and function, semiquantitative estimates of regurgitation severity, and noninvasive hemodynamic measurement of intracardiac pressures (130, 131). Current estimation of PR severity relies on measurement of the ratio of PR jet width to pulmonary annular diameter, as well as an assessment of diastolic flow reversal in the branch PAs 1–2 cm distal to the bifurcation of the main PA (Williams et al., 2002). In 20 pediatric patients who underwent catheterization with contrast pulmonary angiography within 6 months (mean of 1.7 ± 1.6) of echocardiography, the Spearman rank order correlation was 0.95, p <0.001. A clear separation between angiographic grades 0–1+ and 2+–3+ was seen at a color jet/annular ratio of 0.4. A ratio of 0.7 tended to separate angiographic grades 2+ and 3+.

**128** Pulmonary regurgitation associated with severe pulmonary hypertension in a patient with an atrial septal defect. The high frequency (HF) decrescendo diastolic murmur is best heard at the pulmonary artery auscultation area (PA) and begins with a loud $P_2$. Also note the late ejection sound (X) and the short systolic ejection murmur at the pulmonic area related to increased pulmonic flow. A: apical auscultation area; DM: diastolic murmur; SM: systolic murmur. (Adapted from Tavel ME (1972). *Clinical Phonocardiography and External Pulse Recording.* Yearbook Medical Publishers, Chicago.)

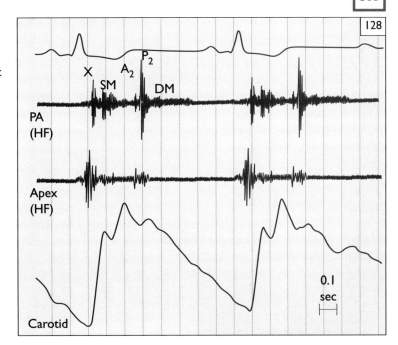

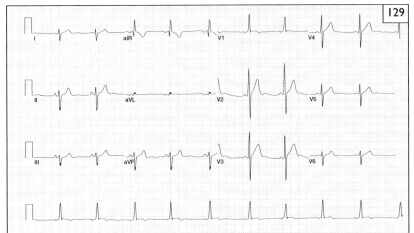

**129** 12-lead electrocardiogram demonstrating findings consistent with pulmonic regurgitation. Note the right axis deviation and R >S in $V_1$ suggesting right ventricular hypertrophy. (Courtesy of Frances DeRook, MD.)

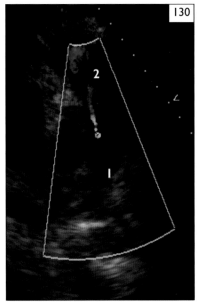

**130** 2D echocardiogram with Doppler color flow mapping displaying the base of the heart in short axis. Pulmonic regurgitation is represented by the orange encoded jet directed from the main pulmonary artery (1) to the right ventricular outflow tract (2).

**131** Continuous wave Doppler interrogation of pulmonic regurgitation jet. Using the modified Bernoulli equation ($P=4V^2$), the pulmonary artery – right ventricular (RV) pressure gradient at end-diastole can be estimated. By adding an estimate of RV end-diastolic pressure (e.g. by assessment of neck veins or inferior vena cava plethora), a noninvasive assessment of pulmonary artery diastolic pressure is obtained. As noted in the text, pulmonary artery systolic pressure is estimated by the peak velocity of the tricuspid regurgitant jet.

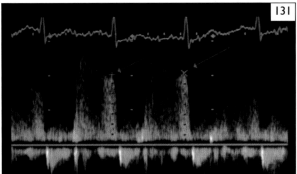

## Cardiac catheterization

Invasive assessment by cardiac catheterization was the original means of obtaining hemodynamic information in pulmonic regurgitation. By borrowing the technique employed in invasive assessment of AR, PR can be scored on a 0–3 point scale following power injection of contrast into the main PA as follows: 0: no reflux of contrast into the RV; 1+ : contrast enters but does not fill the RV; 2+: contrast fills the RV but does not reach the density of contrast in the pulmonary artery; 3+: contrast fills the RV as densely as the PA.

## Medical, surgical, and percutaneous intervention

Mild to moderate PR rarely causes morbidity or mortality. Medical management consists largely of educating the patient in the indications for endocarditis prophylaxis and monitoring for worsening valve dysfunction, progressive RV dilatation, and symptoms and signs of right heart failure.

Severe PR may lead to RV decompensation as noted above. For these patients, medical therapy directed at relief of symptoms includes sodium restriction, diuretic therapy, and digoxin. Traditionally, surgical valve replacement with cadaveric allograft or a porcine bioprosthesis is reserved for patients with refractory right heart failure (Braunwald, 2001). Mechanical prostheses are avoided in these patients because of the excessive risk of thromboembolic complications.

However, in a manner analogous to chronic AR, severe PR can lead insidiously to irreversible RV dilatation and dysfunction (Ebert, 1982; Shimazaki et al., 1984). In the case of adults with remote repair of tetralogy of Fallot and chronic PR, RV dilatation has been linked with an increased risk of sudden death (Marie et al., 1992; Gatzoulis et al., 1995). This has led some investigators to suggest that pulmonary valve replacement be pursued at the earliest stages of RV dilatation. In support of this approach, 25 consecutive adult patients undergoing pulmonary valve replacement were assessed by both pre- and postoperative radionuclide angiography. While there was no statistically significant difference in overall pre- and post-operative RV volumes or ejection fraction (RVEF), 5 of the 10 (50%) patients with a preoperative RVEF >40% had a postoperative RVEF >40%, while only 2 of 15 (13%) patients with a preoperative RVEF <40% had an RVEF >40% postoperatively (Therrien et al., 2002).

An emerging technique is percutaneous insertion of a pulmonary valve. The early experience with a bovine jugular valve was recently reported (Bonhoeffer, 2002). This group manually crimped an 18 mm bovine valve sutured to a platinum stent onto an 18 mm × 4 cm balloon. Placed inside an 18 or 20 French sheath, the device was positioned in the PA and deployed there by withdrawing the sheath and inflating the balloon.

The favorable early results are encouraging. If the percutaneous placement of prosthetic valves proves to be safe and effective, the technique may allow the treatment of patients who currently suffer from severe regurgitation but have comorbidities which preclude open chest surgery. While percutaneous approaches have played a role in stenotic valve lesions for decades, this advance into the treatment of regurgitant lesions represents a new frontier. The indications and patient selection are currently being debated (Khambadkone, 2004). Blazing the way for percutaneous aortic valve replacement, it is expected that this approach has the potential to spare patients open chest surgery (Khambadkone and Bonhoeffer, 2004).

## Case study

A 55-year-old sought help from his local family physician for complaints of excessive sleepiness, dyspnea with minor exertion, and swollen feet and ankles. His symptoms had developed slowly over the preceding 2 years. Over this same time he had gained 20 kg (45 lb), which he attributed to a sudden decrease in physical activity following a knee injury. His medical history was significant for a 60 pack-year smoking history, hypertension, type 2 diabetes mellitus, gout, osteoarthritis, dyslipidemia, and open angle glaucoma. His medications included lisinopril 20 mg daily, glyburide 5 mg twice daily, lovastatin 40 mg at bedtime, allopurinol 300 mg daily, aspirin 81 mg daily, and acetaminophen 1000 mg four times daily.

He had not worked since winning a sizable lottery prize 2 years earlier, but he had previously been employed as a security guard at a nuclear power plant. He was divorced, had two grown children, reported his alcohol consumption as 12 beers per day, and enjoyed watching sports, especially football and auto racing, on television.

On exam, he was an obese man with a plethoric complexion and a short thick neck who had to be awakened in the crowded waiting room. He had mild scleral icterus, palmer erythema, scattered telangiectasia on his face, back, and chest. His blood pressure was 182/94 mmHg (24.3/12.5 kPa) in the left arm and 186/92 mmHg (24.8/12.3 kPa) in the right. His pulse was 84 bpm and regular. His resting room air arterial oxygen saturation by transcutaneous measurement was 82%. His jugular venous pulsations reached the angle of his jaw while sitting up. He had no carotid bruits and brisk upstrokes of both carotid arteries. Examination of the chest disclosed gynecomastia, increased AP diameter, hyperresonance, a prolonged expiratory phase, and mild expiratory wheezing. An RV lift was present as well as a systolic pulsation in the left 2nd intercostal space. $S_1$ was normal; $S_2$ was widely split but not fixed. A 2/6 systolic ejection murmur was audible at the left upper sternal border and a high-pitched, blowing, decrescendo, early diastolic murmur which increased with inspiration was audible along the left sternal border. He had ascites and a tender liver palpable one hand's breath below the costal margin. His testes were small and he had guaic-positive stool. Pitting edema to the knees was present. Cognition and motor function were grossly normal.

ECG revealed sinus rhythm with a tall P wave in lead II, right axis deviation, an R wave greater than S in V1 and low voltage. Chest X-ray suggested hyperinflation, scant peripheral vasculature, and near obliteration of the retrosternal clear space on the lateral film. Abnormalities of his blood chemistries included a direct hyperbilirubinemia, elevated transaminases (alanine aminotransferase [ALT] in excess of aspartate aminotransferase [AST]), a microcytic anemia, and mild thrombocytopenia.

He subsequently underwent endoscopy revealing small esophageal varices, liver biopsy revealing early stage cirrhosis, and measurement of lung volumes and spirometry confirming moderate obstruction of airflow improving with bronchodilators. Polysomnography revealed very brief sleep latency and repeated episodes of obstructive sleep apnea (OSA) with desaturations to the mid 60% range. Transthoracic echocardiography demonstrated an estimated pulmonary artery systolic pressure (PASP) of 80 mmHg (10.7 kPa) moderate-severe PR through a morphologically normal pulmonary valve. The RV was both dilated and thickened. Left-sided cardiac structure and function was normal. The inferior vena cava (IVC) was plethoric and did not collapse with inspiration.

Confronted with unexpectedly grave health problems, he committed to making fundamental changes in his lifestyle. Over the following 2 months he underwent counseling to help him abstain from alcohol and cigarettes, began exercising on a stationary bike for 60 minutes daily, and adopted a vegetarian diet. On his fifth try, he quit smoking. He gave his plasma screen TV set to a nursing home and started volunteering for his town's youth recreation program. He began nasal continuous positive airway pressure ventilation, continuous daytime oxygen supplementation, and inhaled bronchodilators. He lost 22.5 kg (50 lb). On follow-up echocardiography 1 year later, his estimated PASP was 45 mmHg (6.0 kPa), and showed only mild PR and a normal sized RV and IVC.

COMMENTS

This vignette outlines common symptoms and findings of pulmonary hypertension with severe PR. In this case, the pulmonary hypertension was due to a reversible cause, OSA and reactive airway disease. The multisystem nature of valve disease (most disease for that matter) is also evident. In this case, OSA and reactive airway disease produced sequelae involving the cardiovascular, gastrointestinal/hepatic, hematopoietic, and neurologic systems. The case also demonstrates that definitive treatment is not always surgical.

## References

Bonhoeffer P, Boudjemline Y, Qureshi SA, *et al.* (2002). Percutaneous insertion of the pulmonary valve. *Journal of the American College of Cardiology* 39(10):1664–1669.

Braunwald E (2001). Valvular heart disease. In *Heart Disease: A Textbook of Cardiovascular Medicine*. E Braunwald, DP Zipes, P Libby (eds). WB Saunders, Philadelphia, pp.1643–1722.

Ebert PA (1982). Second operations for pulmonary stenosis or insufficiency after repair of tetralogy of Fallot. *American Journal of Cardiology* 50:637–640.

Gatzoulis MA, Till JA, Somervill J, Redington AN (1995). Mechano-electrical interaction in tetralogy of Fallot: QRS prolongation relates to right ventricular size and predicts malignant ventricular arrhythmias and sudden death. *Circulation* 92:231–237.

Khambadkone S, Bonhoeffer P (2004). Nonsurgical pulmonary valve replacement: why, when, and how? *Catheterization and Cardiovascular Interventions* 62(3):401–408.

Marie PY, Marcon F, Brunotte F, *et al.* (1992). Right ventricular overload and induced sustained ventricular tachycardia in operatively 'repaired' tetralogy of Fallot. *American Journal of Cardiology* 69:785–789.

Pouget JM, Kelly C, Pilz C (1967). Congenital absence of the pulmonic valve: report of a case in a 73-year-old man. *American Journal of Cardiology* 19:732–734.

Sayger P, Lewis M, Arcilla R, Ilbawi M (2000). Isolated congenital absence of a single pulmonary valve cusp. *Pediatric Cardiology* 21:487–489.

Sherman SV, Wall MH, Kennedy DJ, Brooker RF, Butterworth J (2001). Do pulmonary artery catheters cause or increase tricuspid or pulmonic valvular regurgitation? *Anesthesia and Analgesia* 92:1117–1122.

Shimazaki Y, Blackstone EH, Kirklin JW (1984). The natural history of isolated congenital pulmonary valve incompetence: surgical implications. *Thoracic and Cardiovascular Surgery* 32:257–259.

Therrien J, Siu SC, McLaughlin PR, Liu PP, Williams WG, Webb GD (2002). Pulmonary valve replacement in adults late after repair of tetralogy of Fallot: are we operating too late? *Journal of the American College of Cardiology* 36(5):1670–1675.

Williams RV, Minich LL, Shaddy RE, Pagotto LT, Tani LY (2002). Comparison of Doppler echocardiography with angiography for determining the severity of pulmonary regurgitation. *American Journal of Cardiology* 89:1438–1441.

# Chapter Thirteen

# Tricuspid Stenosis

## Definition

Obstruction to antegrade flow producing a measurable pressure gradient is considered stenosis. Severity is described in a manner similar to mitral stenosis (MS), as the mean pressure gradient across the valve or the estimated valve area. Most commonly, this is calculated from blood flow velocity measurements by continuous wave Doppler. Mean pressure gradients <5 mmHg (0.7 kPa) are mild, 5–10 mmHg (0.7–1.3 kPa) are considered moderate, and gradients >10 mmHg (1.3 kPa) are considered severe.

## Etiology

The most common cause of tricuspid stenosis (TS) is rheumatic heart disease. Mild TS is present in 10–15% of patients with rheumatic heart disease, but clinically significant TS is quite rare, occurring in only 3–5%. Rheumatic TS without involvement of the mitral or the aortic valve is extremely uncommon. Other causes are very rare and include infective endocarditis with bulky vegetations, carcinoid syndrome, congenital tricuspid atresia, Fabry's disease, Whipple's disease,

and methysergide toxicity. Right atrial (RA) tumors (**132**) and thrombus (**133–135**) may produce the functional equivalent of TS (Waller *et al.*, 1995). Finally, trauma from instrumentation or long-term indwelling devices may result in TS.

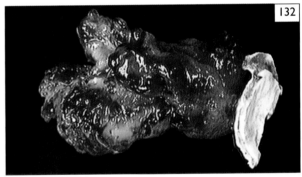

**132** Gross pathology specimen of a resected atrium myxoma. Note the polypoid morphology and the cut surface attachment point. (Courtesy of Tom Farrell, MD.)

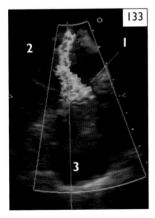

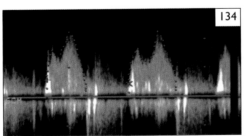

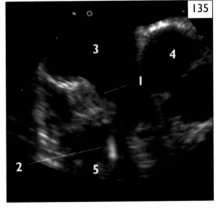

**133–135** Functional tricuspid stenosis. **133** Doppler color flow map of the right ventricular (RV) inflow demonstrating aliasing (high velocity) antegrade flow through the mitral valve (1). 2: right ventricle; 3: right atrium. **134** Continuous wave Doppler imaging of RV inflow revealing an estimated mean pressure gradient of 9 mmHg (1.2 kPa). **135** Transesophageal imaging of the same patient revealing that the obstruction is due to thrombus (1) adherent to a pacer lead (2). This patient was hypercoaguable due to a prothrombin gene mutation. 3: right atrium; 4: aortic valve; 5: right ventricle.

## Pathophysiology

Obstruction of flow across the tricuspid valve serves to limit increases in cardiac output and hence exercise tolerance. In addition, mean gradients as low as 5 mmHg (0.7 kPa) result in elevation of RA pressure, especially during expiration. This increase in pressure leads to RA enlargement and is transmitted to the systemic venous circulation. Since diastole is disproportionately shortened with increasing heart rate, tachycardia can produce dramatic increases in the pressure gradient by shortening the time available for antegrade transvalvular flow.

## Clinical presentation

### SYMPTOMS

Most patients with rheumatic TS are symptomatic from coexisting left-sided valvular lesions. Common symptoms attributable specifically to TS include fatigue, right upper quadrant discomfort from hepatic congestion and stretch of the hepatic capsule, abdominal bloating, and lower extremity edema without orthopnea. In some cases, anorexia, nausea, vomiting, and eructation caused by portal venous hypertension may be prominent (Hillis et al., 1992). Some patients may notice abnormal pulsations in their neck caused by dramatic jugular a waves.

### SIGNS

Careful physical exam may reveal signs of systemic venous hypertension. These signs include evidence of increased central venous pressure (136) with prominent a wave pulsations, distension of the veins of the upper arm, and even of the dorsum of the extended hand. This pressure will dramatically increase with sustained compression of the central abdomen as blood is redistributed from the liver and gut (i.e. hepatojugular reflux). Other signs of elevated systemic venous hypertension include weight gain, ascites, hepatomegaly which may be massive, and peripheral edema ranging from ankle swelling to anasarca. Corresponding to the jugular a wave, a presystolic hepatic pulsation may be appreciated.

On precordial examination, cardiac percussion may reveal that the heart is enlarged to the right, in some cases reaching the midclavicular line. Palpation may

disclose a diastolic thrill, most prominent during inspiration, felt at the left lower sternal border. Auscultation is made challenging by the frequent coexistence of mitral and aortic stenosis in patients with rheumatic disease. Since the tricuspid leaflets are closing from a nearly fully open position and because they have often lost their pliability, $S_1$ is often increased in intensity. If coexisting left-sided valve disease has caused pulmonary hypertension, $P_2$ may be increased in intensity as well. Although difficult to appreciate in the presence of coexistent mitral stenosis, an opening snap 60–80 msec following $P_2$ may be heard, followed in turn by a soft, high-pitched, diamond-shaped, diastolic murmur best heard at the left fourth intercostal space and accentuated by maneuvers which increase venous return, the simplest of which is inspiration. Assigning this murmur to the tricuspid valve is based on its location at the left lower sternal border (in contrast to the diastolic murmur of MS at the apex), the higher, softer, and shorter nature of TS in comparison to MS, and the absence of orthopnea and crackles on lung exam which commonly accompany MS (Braunwald, 2001).

### LABORATORY FINDINGS

#### Electrocardiography

The electrocardiogram (ECG) may provide evidence of RA enlargement, manifest as a P wave exceeding 2.5 mm in limb lead II or 1.5 mm in $V_1$ (137). As a result of the increased distance traveled from the sinoatrial node to the atrioventricular node, first degree atrioventricular block may be evident. In advanced disease, the distortion of the atrial tissue is likely to trigger atrial fibrillation.

#### Chest radiography

The chest radiograph may reveal cardiomegaly with RA prominence. The superior vena cava may appear widened and, under fluoroscopy, may demonstrate presystolic pulsations. If MS is present as well, biatrial enlargement will also be seen with accompanying evidence of pulmonary vascular and interstitial congestion. When calcification accompanies valve stenosis, it may be evident on chest radiography (138).

**136** Distended jugular vein (arrow) in a 32-year-old male who developed severe tricuspid stenosis of a bioprosthetic valve. (Reprinted from Battle RW, Galvin JM (2001). Images in clinical medicine. Critical tricuspid stenosis with severe venous hypertension. *New England Journal of Medicine* **344**(3):196–197. With permission. Copyright Massachusetts Medical Society. All rights reserved.)

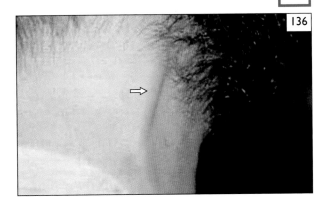

**137** 12-lead electrocardiogram from a patient with confirmed tricuspid stenosis. P wave amplitude is prominent in lead II but does not make the criterion of 2.5 mm. Right bundle branch block is evident.

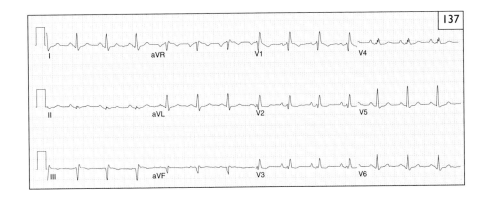

**138** Anteroposterior chest radiograph from the patient described in **136**. Calcification of the three tricuspid leaflets within the bioprosthetic valve stents are faintly visible (epicardial pacing wires are also apparent). (Reprinted from Battle RW, Galvin JM (2001). Images in clinical medicine. Critical tricuspid stenosis with severe venous hypertension. *New England Journal of Medicine* **344**(3):196–197. With permission. Copyright Massachusetts Medical Society. All rights reserved.)

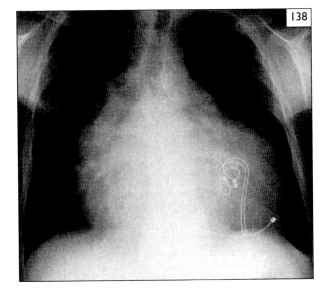

## Echocardiography

Echocardiography is the most commonly utilized imaging modality in the evaluation of tricuspid valve disease. Transthoracic 2D imaging can provide information about the general morphology and motion of the valve. Typically, the valve leaflets appear thickened, exhibit greatly limited mobility, and assume a dome-like shape in diastole. Right and left ventricular function and any associated congenital anomalies can also be assessed. Transesophageal imaging can provide a much more detailed view of tricuspid valve morphology including possible evidence of valvular vegetations. Echocardiographic Doppler interrogation typically demonstrates prolonged, high velocity antegrade flow through the tricuspid orifice (**139**). Doppler ultrasound may also display flow reversal in the inferior vena cava during atrial systole. This corresponds to the presystolic hepatic pulsation noted on physical exam (Hillis *et al.*, 1992).

## Cardiac catheterization

Direct measurement of intracardiac pressures has been the traditional method of confirming and quantitating TS. However, improvements in echocardiography have relegated invasive assessments to cases in which there is a discrepancy between clinical and echocardiographic data, or when coronary angiography is indicated prior to surgical valve repair. Carefully performed echocardiographic assessments generally provide similar results to invasive measurements (**140**).

## Medical management

As seen in many of the other valve lesions, patients may tolerate TS for decades before they develop lifestyle limiting symptoms. However, if the degree of stenosis is severe, patients eventually exhaust their ability to compensate and develop the symptoms described above. Throughout the course, the general considerations of endocarditis prophylaxis, rheumatic fever prophylaxis (if indicated), and rate control and anticoagulation for atrial fibrillation apply. Once symptoms of right-sided failure appear, heart rate slowing to maximize diastolic filling time, sodium restriction, and judicious diuretic use are helpful, but ultimately the problem requires a mechanical solution.

## Percutaneous and surgical intervention

The criteria for intervention include right-sided heart failure and a mean diastolic pressure gradient >5 mmHg (0.7 kPa) and an estimated tricuspid orifice of <2.0 cm$^2$ (Kirklin and Barratt-Boyes, 1993). Current options range from balloon valvuloplasty to open valvotomy or tricuspid valve replacement with a large bioprosthesis. A tissue valve is usually chosen because of the very high risk of thromboembolism associated with a mechanical prosthesis in this position. Valve replacement avoids the risk of severe tricuspid regurgitation posed by valvuloplasty, but with the trade-off of higher procedural risk.

In rare instances, generally limited to pediatric congenital heart disease, neither valve repair nor replacement is possible. In these cases, consideration of extracardiac homograft connections, such as the placement of an aortic homograft between the RA and the right ventricle must be considered (Al-Halees and Al-Fadley, 1997).

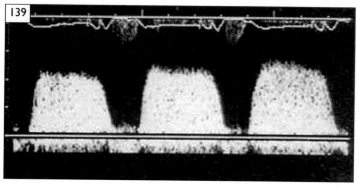

**139** A continuous wave Doppler velocity profile across the tricuspid valve shown in **137**. The mean transvalvular pressure gradient calculated from this velocity was 26 mmHg (3.5 kPa). (Reprinted from Battle RW, Galvin JM (2001). Images in clinical medicine. Critical tricuspid stenosis with severe venous hypertension. *New England Journal of Medicine* **344**(3):196–197. With permission. Copyright Massachusetts Medical Society. All rights reserved.)

**140** Simultaneous right atrial (RA) and right ventricular (RV) pressure recordings from the same 32-year-old male described in **136**. The mean RA pressure was 37 mmHg (4.9 kPa) and the mean diastolic pressure gradient between two chambers was 24 mmHg (3.2 kPa). (Reprinted from Battle RW, Galvin JM (2001). Images in clinical medicine. Critical tricuspid stenosis with severe venous hypertension. *New England Journal of Medicine* **344**(3):196–197. With permission. Copyright Massachusetts Medical Society. All rights reserved.)

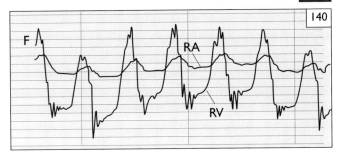

## Case study

A 60-year-old woman visited her nurse practitioner with complaints of progressive shortness of breath and ankle edema. Three months earlier she had noticed shortness of breath when stacking hay in the family's barn. Approximately 2 months earlier she noticed mild ankle edema by late afternoon, and dyspnea when carrying wet laundry from the basement to the back yard clothesline. Beginning 2 weeks earlier, she noticed persistent ankle edema and increasing fatigue. On several occasions she experienced sudden onset of shortness of breath at rest that gradually abated over a few days. She denied chest pressure or heaviness and denied fever or chills.

Her past history was notable only for mild obesity and several relatively minor traumatic injuries. Her only medication was calcium carbonate twice daily. She worked early mornings, evenings, and weekends on her family's dairy farm and four 10-hour days per week as an emergency room nurse. She had never smoked and consumed approximately three glasses of wine per week. Her family history was significant only for unusual longevity.

On exam, she was a fit looking woman, who appeared younger than her stated age. Her blood pressure was 135/65 mmHg (18/8.7 kPa) and her pulse was 100 bpm and irregularly irregular. Her estimated right atrial pressure was 12 cm of $H_2O$. The carotids were free of bruits and demonstrated normal upstrokes. No crackles or wheezes were heard during auscultation of her chest. She had no right ventricular heave, her point of maximal intensity (PMI) was not displaced, and she had no thrills. Her heart sounds were irregularly irregular and tachycardic, with a soft $S_1$ and a low-pitched diastolic murmur heard at the left lower sternal border. Her liver was enlarged with a span by percussion of 15 cm. Pitting edema to the midshin was present bilaterally.

ECG confirmed atrial fibrillation with a rapid ventricular response. Blood chemistry was notable for a normochromic normocytic anemia and an elevated erythrocyte sedimentation rate of 90 mm/hour.

The patient was started on warfarin for stroke prophylaxis and metoprolol for control of ventricular rate. Auscultation at a heart rate of 62 bpm revealed a low-pitched extra heart sound in early diastole.

Echocardiography performed 3 weeks later was technically limited due to poor echocardiographic windows and outdated equipment, but the findings included a dilated RA, high velocity flow across the tricuspid valve by Doppler interrogation, and a distended inferior vena cava. Two weeks later, a transesophageal echocardiogram was performed which revealed a 3 cm × 5 cm irregularly shaped right atrial mass on a stalk attached near the tricuspid annulus. Pelvic exam, liver chemistries, and computed tomography of the chest, abdomen, and pelvis revealed no abnormalities.

After consultatations with cardiology, oncology, and cardiothoracic surgery at a tertiary academic medical center, she underwent 'minimally invasive' surgery by 'L'-shaped sternotomy, atriotomy, and excision of a 3.3 cm × 4.8 cm atrial myxoma.

The patient had an uneventful recovery and was discharged on postoperative day 3. Two months later, she was in sinus rhythm and her right atrial dimension had returned to normal size. Four months later, after she had confirmed a regular rhythm by daily pulse check, she stopped her warfarin. She returned to 4 am milking and her emergency room nursing responsibilities.

## COMMENTS

This case study portrays a previously healthy woman who develops a right atrial myxoma which behaves physiologically as TS. The common sequelae of atrial fibrillation and right heart failure are included. The limitation of transthoracic echocardiography and the value of a transesophageal approach are demonstrated. Some surgeons, in the hopes of less postoperative discomfort and a faster recovery, employ an 'L'-shaped sternotomy incision.

## References

Al-Halees Z, Al-Fadley F (1997). Extracardiac right atrium to right ventricle homograft for uncorrectable tricuspid valve disease. *Annals of Thoracic Surgery* **63**(6):1794–1796.

Braunwald E (2001). Valvular heart disease. In: *Heart Disease: A Textbook of Cardiovascular Medicine*. E Braunwald, DP Zipes, P Libby (eds). WB Saunders, Philadelphia, ch 46, pp. 1643–1722.

Hillis LD, Lange RA, Wells PJ, Winniford MD (1992). Valvular heart disease. In: *Manual of Clinical Problems in Cardiology*, 4th edn. Little, Brown and Company, Boston, pp. 230–237.

Kirklin JW, Barratt-Boyes BG (1993). *Tricuspid valve disease*. In: Cardiac Surgery, 2nd edn. JW Kirklin, BF Barratt-Boyes (eds). Churchill-Livingstone, New York, pp. 589–608.

Waller BF, Howard J, Fess S (1995). Pathology of tricuspid valve stenosis and pure tricuspid regurgitation: part I. *Clinical Cardiology* **18**:97–102.

# Chapter Fourteen

# Tricuspid Regurgitation

### Definition

Tricuspid regurgitation (TR) refers to retrograde flow through the right-sided atrioventricular valve during systole. Trivial amounts are seen in the majority of healthy adults. As in all regurgitant valve lesions, the severity is most commonly graded on a semiquantitative scale. This scale begins at 0 (none), followed by 'trivial' (physiologic), 1+ (mild), 2+ (moderate), 3+ (moderate–severe), and 4+ (severe).

Alternatively, using careful 2D and echo Doppler measurements and formulae beyond the scope of this handbook, TR can be graded quantitatively. These volumetric descriptions of regurgitant lesions include the effective regurgitant orifice (ERO) and the regurgitant volume ($V_{regurg}$). Based on the threshold of regurgitation necessary for reversal of venous flow (hepatic for TR and pulmonary for mitral regurgitation [MR]), an ERO of 40 $mm^2$ has been proposed as the cut-off, above which both TR and MR should be considered severe (Tribouilloy *et al.*, 2002). Interestingly, this corresponds to different regurgitant volumes. The minimal regurgitant volume producing venous flow reversal is 60 ml/beat in MR and 45 ml/beat in TR, due to the difference in the ventriculoatrial pressure gradient (the driving gradient) on the right and left sides of the heart.

### Etiology

As discussed in the case of MR, a practical and common classification scheme is to divide causes into functional and structural. Structural causes can be further divided into congenital and acquired. Most cases of TR are functional; they arise from distortion of the right ventricle (RV) or annulus due to pulmonary hypertension exceeding 55 mmHg (7.3 kPa) (**141, 142**), RV infarct, or dilated

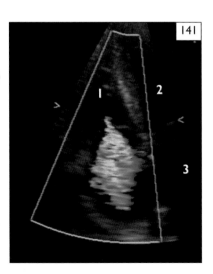
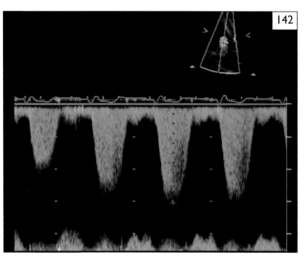

**141, 142** Moderate tricuspid regurgitation (TR) with pulmonary hypertension. **141** Doppler color imaging in the apical 4-chamber view, demonstrating probably moderate TR in a heart transplant patient. 1: right ventricle; 2: left ventricle; 3: left atrium. **142** Continuous wave Doppler interrogation of TR jet velocity revealing an estimated right ventricular/ right atrial peak instantaneous gradient of 38 mmHg (5.1 kPa). This number is added to estimated right atrial pressure to arrive at an estimate of pulmonary artery systolic pressure.

cardiomyopathy (Bonow *et al.*, 1998). TR resulting from acquired structural abnormalities of the valve occurs in rheumatic valvulitis, infective endocarditis, carcinoid syndrome, rheumatoid arthritis, radiation therapy, Marfan syndrome, myxomatous valve disease, congenital heart disease and, possibly, to anorexigen use (Waller *et al.*, 1995).

### Pathophysiology

Analogous to left-sided atrioventricular regurgitation, the venous circulation (in this case, systemic venous), atrial function, ventricular function, and cardiac output are all influenced by a severely leaking tricuspid valve. Viewing the process sequentially beginning with the atrium, the regurgitant volume increases right atrial (RA) pressure in inverse proportion to RA compliance. Acutely, the RA is poorly compliant and nondilated. In this circumstance, small regurgitant volumes are translated into significant increases in pressure and are manifest on RA tracings as c-v waves. This raises mean RA pressure and serves to impair systemic venous return. RA pressure may be dramatically elevated in the context of pulmonary hypertension. As a result, venous congestion develops and is manifest by the clinical symptoms and signs described below.

Over time, the RA gradually dilates and becomes more compliant. While RA pressure may fall somewhat, the dilatation is accompanied by other physiologic derangements including a diathesis towards atrial fibrillation and thrombus formation. This may lead to pulmonary emboli or, in the 20–25% of the population possessing a patent foramen ovale, paradoxical systemic emboli.

The RV is burdened with a volume load. It is obliged to pump not only the systemic venous blood returning from the vena cava and the coronary sinus, but also the TR volume. Initially, the RV maintains forward cardiac output by increasing total stroke volume (regurgitant volume + net forward stroke volume). This adaptation is facilitated by the increased preload of the regurgitant volume and the diminished afterload of a leaky valve. This process of moderate dilatation is similar to the eccentric hypertrophy of chronic aortic regurgitation (AR). However, if severe, decompensation eventually occurs. As RV systolic function fails, it becomes unable to achieve its normal end-diastolic volume and pathologic dilatation develops. The annular dilatation in turn increases any functional component of TR (**143, 144**).

From the perspective of cardiac output, the preferential ejection of blood into the low pressure RA and, in end-stage disease, the failing systolic function, result in a greatly diminished cardiac output. Since the left heart can only pump what is delivered from the right side, any impairment in right-sided cardiac output is accompanied by equal impairment in systemic cardiac output.

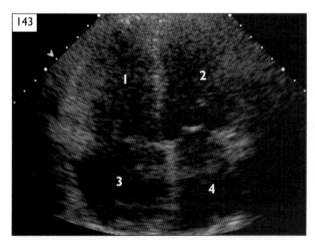

**143** Apical 4-chamber echocardiographic view of a patient with severe tricuspid regurgitation. Note the dilatation of the right ventricle and right atrium resulting from the chronic volume burden. 1: right ventricle; 2: left ventricle; 3: right atrium; 4: left atrium.

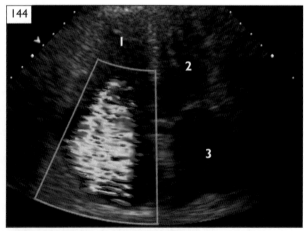

**144** Doppler color flow imaging of the tricuspid regurgitation jet in severe tricuspid regurgitation. 1: right ventricle; 2: left ventricle; 3: left atrium.

## Clinical presentation

SYMPTOMS

Mild and moderate degrees of TR are very well tolerated. However, severe TR, especially when accompanied by pulmonary hypertension, often produces symptoms of fatigue, peripheral edema, anorexia, nausea, vomiting, eructation, and right upper quadrant discomfort. Neck and eyeball pulsations are sometimes reported by patients (Allen and Naylor, 1985).

SIGNS

Common general physical findings include cachexia, jaundice, eccymoses, severe peripheral edema, ascites, and tender, pulsatile hepatomegaly. One sign distinguishing TR from tricuspid stenosis is this more pulsatile venous hypertension resulting from ventricular, rather than atrial, contraction. With pulmonary hypertension, cyanosis may occur from right-to-left shunting across a patent foramen ovale.

Specific cardiovascular findings include distended neck veins with a regurgitation-induced c-v wave; an RV lift arising from increased RV stroke volume; extension of the heart into the right chest detected by percussion; a soft $S_1$ related to failure of tricuspid valve coaptation; a loud $P_2$ in pulmonary hypertension; a right-sided $S_3$ associated with RV dilatation; a blowing, holosystolic, regurgitant murmur heard best at the left lower sternal border and accentuated by inspiration (Carvallo's sign); and a low-pitched, diastolic rumble of increased antegrade flow across the tricuspid valve.

LABORATORY FINDINGS

*Electrocardiography*

Electrocardiographic (ECG) findings may include atrial fibrillation, RA enlargement, right axis deviation, RV hypertrophy, or incomplete right bundle branch block (**145**).

*Chest radiography*

In functional TR, the RV may be enlarged on chest radiography. Elevated RA pressure may produce distension of the azygos vein and bilateral pleural effusions. (Recall that the bronchial veins are part of the systemic venous circulation.)

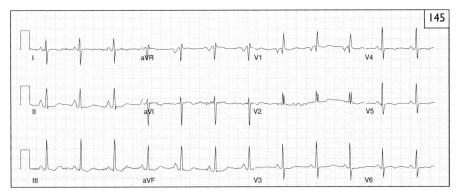

**145** 12-lead electrocardiogram of a patient with severe tricuspid regurgitation and severe pulmonary hypertension (70 mmHg [9.3 kPa] maximum instantaneous gradient by Doppler). This tracing demonstrates right atrial abnormality (note the P wave amplitude in II) and right ventricular hypertrophy. Unexplained left atrial abnormality is also evident. (Courtesy of Frances DeRook, MD.)

*Echocardiography*
Echocardiography is the cornerstone of laboratory evaluation of TR (**146**). Transthoracic 2D imaging can often provide sufficient anatomic detail to elucidate the mechanism of the valvular leak. In some cases, transesophageal echocardiography (TEE), by virtue of its higher frequency transducer with improved resolution, is necessary to characterize the specific anatomic derangement responsible for the regurgitation. Doppler color flow mapping, by displaying the degree to which regurgitant flow penetrates the RA, provides a semiquantitative measure of TR. Using pulsed and continuous wave Doppler interrogation of intracavitary flow, quantitative (volumetric) assessment of TR is possible. This is done by comparing the stroke volume (cross-sectional area of valve × distance traveled by a red blood cell per cardiac cycle) of the tricuspid valve and the pulmonic valve. The difference represents regurgitant volume.

To avoid underestimation of TR severity which accompanies difficulty in detecting the regurgitant flow, investigators have experimented with augmenting the ultrasound signal by injecting mixtures of 10% air/90% saline or 10% air/10% blood/80% saline. This relatively simple bedside maneuver significantly improved the correlation of Doppler-based estimates with Swan-Ganz catheter-based measurements of pulmonary artery systolic pressure. Based on studies of 20 patients, the correlation coefficient (r) was 0.64 for standard measurement, 0.86 for the agitated air/saline mixture, and 0.92 for the agitated air/blood/saline mixture (Jeon *et al.*, 2002).

Additional information provided by echocardiography includes RV size, RV function, and estimates of RA pressure based on plethora of the inferior vena cava.

*Cardiac catheterization*
Invasive hemodynamic measurements obtained by right heart catheterization can also be used to assess TR. Pressure tracings are characterized by a prominent c-v wave (**147**). As a limited 'rule of thumb', an RV pressure >60 mmHg (8 kPa) suggests a functional origin to the TR, while an RV pressure <40 mmHg (5.3 kPa) suggests an organic basis for the TR.

**Natural history**
While many patients with normal left ventricular (LV) function tolerate TR without difficulty, in those patients with LV systolic dysfunction, TR appears to portend a worse prognosis. A recent retrospective study of 1421 consecutive patients with ejection fraction (EF) ≤0.35 revealed that the relative risk of death over a mean follow-up period of 1 year was

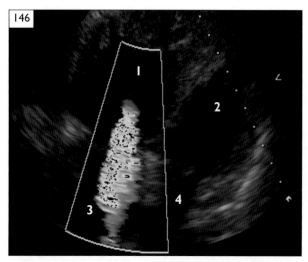

**146** 2D echocardiogram with Doppler color flow mapping displaying the heart from an apical view. Note the right ventricle (1) is nearly equal in size to the left ventricle (2) (normally it is <2/3 of the area) and observe the large jet of tricuspid regurgitant flow. 3: right atrium; 4: left atrium.

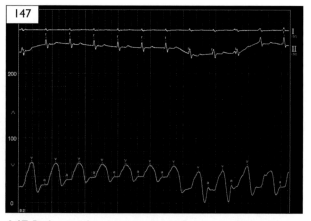

**147** Right atrial pressure tracing from a patient with severe tricuspid regurgitation. Note the prominent c-v wave.

1.55 for severe TR (Koelling *et al.*, 2002). Other investigators have suggested that secondary TR may be an independent predictor of cardiac cachexia and protein-losing enteropathy (Ajayi *et al.*, 1999).

### Medical management

Patients with normal pulmonary pressures do not generally require surgery, even if the TR is severe (Braunwald, 2001). However, in the presence of pulmonary hypertension, the hemodynamic consequences are much more pronounced and often do require surgical intervention, unless the underlying cause of pulmonary hypertension can be addressed (e.g. balloon valvotomy for mitral stenosis). In the case of functional TR due to LV systolic failure, the full armamentarium of heart failure therapy must be considered. This includes pharmacologic treatment with diuretics, angiotensin-converting enzyme inhibitors, digoxin, beta-blockers, and spironolactone. In addition to valve or annular surgery, consideration should be given to volume reduction surgery (e.g. Dor procedure) and resynchronization therapy with biventricular pacemakers (Trichon and O'Connor, 2002).

### Surgical intervention

Functional TR generally responds well to restoration of normal annular size by surgical annuloplasty

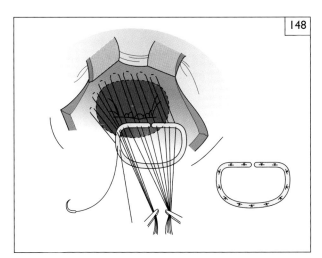

**148** Insertion of an annuloplasty ring. (Adapted from Galloway AC, Colvin SB, Baumann FG, *et al.* (1988). Current concepts of mitral valve reconstruction for mitral insufficiency. *Circulation* **78**:1087–1098.)

(Pellegrini *et al.*, 1992) (**148**). While many centers use flexible rings, rigid rings appear to produce acceptable results as well. Surgeons at Mie University in Japan have reported the results of 45 patients with TR secondary to mitral valve disease in whom a Carpentier–Edwards rigid ring annuloplasty was performed between 1985 and 1996 and followed for a mean of 96.7 ± 48.5 months (Onada *et al.*, 2000). Thirty-nine (86.6%) were in NYHA functional class III or IV. Actuarial survival at 10 years was 68.3%. TR was limited to 2+ or less in all survivors.

When TR is the only abnormality (isolated TR), the decision to proceed with open heart surgery is controversial. A recent retrospective review of 15 consecutive patients (12 with rheumatic disease) undergoing isolated tricuspid valve replacement between 1984 and 1996 found evidence of poor short- and long-term outcomes. Median survival was 1.2 years. Follow-up found 20% died within 30 days and 60% were deceased by 3 years. Anasarca was the only predictor of short-term mortality. Anemia, rheumatic heart disease, previous stroke, and previous mitral valve disease were predictors of long-term mortality (Mangoni *et al.*, 2001). Other investigators retrospectively studying the results of tricuspid valve surgery (repair or replacement) in 12 patients operated on between 1979 and 1998 found evidence of statistically significant reductions in RV end-diastolic and end-systolic volumes, as well as increases in RVEF during a mean follow-up of 130 ± 63 days following surgery (Mukherjee *et al.*, 2000).

Cases of rheumatic heart disease in which TR is associated with commissural fusion may be treated with open valvotomy and ring annuloplasty (Duran, 1994). Morphologically abnormal valves generally require replacement. As noted in earlier chapters, on the right side of the heart where the thrombotic risk of mechanical valves is greater and the durability of tissue valves is better, a tissue valve is generally preferred. In this position, a large porcine bioprosthesis is often selected.

In intravenous drug-related infective endocarditis, aggressive intravenous antibiotics with staged excision and valve replacement 6–9 months later reduces the risk of prosthetic valve infection. In view of the high rate of recurrent drug use and relatively low rates of subsequent right heart failure, some centers have advocated simple tricuspid valve excision (Arbulu *et al.*, 1991).

## Case study

A 72-year-old man went to the emergency room for intolerable fatigue, shortness of breath, loss of appetite, and lower extremity edema. He had no supplemental health insurance, distrusted the medical profession, had no personal physician, and lived alone in a cabin without electricity. Because he quickly became irritated when pressed for details, the particulars of his history remained unknown. However, it seemed that his symptoms had been slowly developing over the past 5 years. He denied any episodes of chest pain, but had had 'spells' of nausea and diaphoresis and epigastric discomfort on many occasions. He had no previously diagnosed health problems to his recollection and no prior visits to this hospital. He took no medications.

He had never been married, had no children, and no known living siblings. He had worked as a logger, trucker, roofer, and hunting guide earlier in life and currently supported himself on a small pension and by hunting and trapping. He chewed tobacco but quit smoking 15 years previously. He had never drunk alcohol.

On exam he was an unkempt, irascible, thin man in mild respiratory distress. His blood pressure was 155/88 mmHg (20.7/11.7 kPa) in both arms, with a resting heart rate of 94 bpm. His respiratory rate was 22 and his oxygen saturation was 88% on room air. His jugular venous pulsations were seen 9 cm above the angle of Louis, with a prominent c-v wave. A left carotid bruit was present. The upstroke of the right carotid was brisk. He had wet sounding inspiratory crackles 1/2 of the way up both lung fields, with bronchial breath sounds and dullness to percussion at the bases. His point of maximal intensity (PMI) was displaced to the 6th intercostal space in the anterior axillary line. An $S_3$ was palpable. He had an RV lift. His heart sounds were regular with a soft $S_1$ and a paradoxically split $S_2$, with both a right-and left-sided $S_3$. A 1/6 decrescendo diastolic murmur was present at the left upper sternal border, and a 3/6 holosystolic murmur, increasing with inspiration, was heard at the left lower sternal border. His liver was pulsating four fingerbreadths beneath the right costal margin. He had ascites and pitting edema to the level of both knees. Reduced visual, olfactory, and gustatory sensation were present along with impaired vibration sense in his feet.

The initial laboratory work revealed hyperglycemia, an elevated serum urea nitrogen (BUN) and creatinine, and hyponatremia. 12-lead ECG showed sinus rhythm with severe 1st degree atrioventricular block (PR interval 360 msec), P waves consistent with biatrial enlargement, and a left bundle branch block pattern. He was admitted to the hospital. An echocardiogram later that day showed a dilated LV with severe systolic dysfunction. The anterior and inferior walls were akinetic and thin. The remaining walls were hypokinetic. The estimated ejection fraction was 20%. The RV was thickened, with an estimated pulmonary artery systolic pressure (PASP) of 65 mmHg (8.7 kPa). There was mild-moderate MR and moderate-severe TR. The inferior vena cava was distended and did not collapse with a sniff.

The patient voiced his intent to leave against medical advice, but was persuaded to stay by a nurse whose family the patient regarded highly. He was diuresed and started on insulin, an angiotensin-converting enzyme (ACE) inhibitor, a beta-blocker, and digoxin on consecutive days. A 24-hour thallium myocardial perfusion study showed no evidence of viability of the anterior and inferior walls, a result consistent with the thin walls seen by echo. He was felt to have advanced ischemic heart disease, complicated by pulmonary hypertension and severe TR. By his eighth hospital day he had achieved normovolemia, his renal function had improved, and he was able to both test his blood sugar and self-administer insulin. He was discharged with support from visiting nurses for continued upward titration of his beta-blocker and ACE inhibitor. Three months later he had improved but still had class III heart failure. Spironolactone was added for aldosterone blockade. A repeat echocardiogram showed diastolic MR and TR attributed to the long PR interval, and evidence of RV and LV dyssynchrony. His ejection fraction had improved to 30% and his systolic MR and TR persisted. He then underwent placement of a biventricular pacemaker and implantable cardio-verter device with Doppler-guided optimization of his programmed AV and RV–LV intervals. With this therapy he improved to NYHA class II heart failure. A follow-up echo revealed improvement in both his MR and TR and a decrease in his estimated PASP to 35 mmHg (4.7 kPa).

## COMMENTS

This vignette portrays the common symptoms and findings of an individual with diabetes and ischemic heart disease. His poor LV systolic function led to pulmonary venous hypertension followed by pulmonary arterial hypertension and functional TR. Aggressive pharmacologic and cardiac resynchronization therapy of his heart failure lead to dramatic improvement in his TR.

## References

Ajayi AA, Adigun AQ, Ojofeitimi EO, *et al.* (1999). Anthropomorphic evaluation of cachexia in chronic congestive heart failure: the role of tricuspid regurgitation. *International Journal of Cardiology* 71:79–84.

Allen SJ, Naylor D (1985). Pulsation of the eyeballs in tricuspid regurgitation. *Canadian Medical Association Journal* 133:119–120.

Arbulu A, Holmes RJ, Asfaw I (1991). Tricuspid valvulectomy without replacement. Twenty years' experience. *Journal of Thoracic and Cardiovascular Surgery* 102(6):917–922.

Bonow RO, Carabello B, de Leon AC Jr, *et al.* (1998). ACC/AHA guidelines for the management of patients with valvular heart disease: a report of the American College of Cardiology/American Heart Association Task Force on practice guidelines (Committee on Management of Patients with Valvular Heart Disease). *Journal of the American College of Cardiology* 32:1486–1588.

Braunwald E (2001). Valvular heart disease. In: *Heart Disease: A Textbook of Cardiovascular Medicine.* E Braunwald, DP Zipes, P Libby (eds). WB Saunders, Philadelphia, ch 46, pp. 1643–1722.

Duran CM (1994). Tricuspid valve surgery revisited. *Journal of Cardiac Surgery* 9:242–247.

Jeon D, Luo H, Iwami T, *et al.* (2002). The usefulness of a 10% air-10% blood-80% saline mixture for contrast echocardiography: Doppler measurement of pulmonary artery systolic pressure. *Journal of the American College of Cardiology* 39(1):124–129.

Koelling TM, Aaronson KD, Cody RJ, Bach DS, Armstrong WF (2002). Prognostic significance of mitral regurgitation and tricuspid regurgitation in patients with left ventricular systolic dysfunction. *American Heart Journal* 144(3):524–529.

Mangoni AA, DiSalvo TG, Vlahakes GJ, Polanczyk CA, Fifer MA (2001). Outcome following isolated tricuspid valve replacement. *European Journal of Cardiothoracic Surgery* 19(1):68–73.

Mukherjee D, Nader S, Olano A, Garcia MJ, Griffin BP (2000). Improvement in right ventricular systolic function after surgical correction of isolated tricuspid regurgitation. *Journal of the American Society of Echocardiography* 13(7):650–654.

Onada K, Yasuda F, Takao M, *et al.* (2000). Long-term follow-up after Carpentier-Edwards ring annuloplasty for tricuspid regurgitation. *Annals of Thoracic Surgery* 70(3): 796–799.

Pellegrini A, Columbo T, Donatelli E, *et al.* (1992). Evaluation and treatment of secondary tricuspid insufficiency. *European Journal of Cardiothoracic Surgery* 6:288–296.

Tribouilloy CM, Enriquez-Sarano M, Capps MA, Bailey KR, Tajik AJ (2002). Contrasting effect of similar effective regurgitant orifice area in mitral and tricuspid regurgitation: a quantitative Doppler echocardiographic study. *Journal of the American Society of Echocardiography* 15(9):958–965.

Trichon BH, O'Connor CM (2002). Secondary mitral and tricuspid regurgitation accompanying left ventricular systolic dysfunction: is it important, and how is it treated? (editorial). *American Heart Journal* 144(3):373–376.

Waller BF, Howard J, Fess S (1995). Pathology of tricuspid valve stenosis and pure tricuspid regurgitation: part III. *Clinical Cardiology* 18:225–230.

# Chapter Fifteen

# Mixed Single Valve Disease

### Aortic stenosis and aortic regurgitation

PATHOPHYSIOLOGY

Aortic valves demonstrating both obstruction and incompetence present a special problem. If either is trivial or mild, it contributes little to the clinical manifestation or management of the dominant valve dysfunction. However, if both are moderate or worse, then the left ventricle (LV) is burdened with simultaneous pressure and volume loads. The concentric LV hypertrophy which develops in response to aortic stenosis (AS) renders the ventricle less compliant and hence disadvantaged in coping with the volume load of aortic regurgitation (AR) (Bonow *et al.*, 1998).

CLINICAL PRESENTATION

Because of the physiology described above, symptoms and physical exam findings may appear with seemingly moderate individual valve lesions. The hemodynamic assessment is also modified by the presence of mixed valve disease. Pressure gradients across a stenotic aortic valve will be augmented by the increased flow accompanying regurgitation. Thus, estimates of severity of stenosis based solely on pressure gradients must be avoided. In addition, calculation of valve area based on invasive hemodynamic data is unreliable and will likely overestimate AS, because Fick and thermodilution estimates of cardiac output measure net forward flow only (not total transvalvular flow). In cases of mixed AR and AS, quantitative echocardiographic estimates of valve area (AVA) and effective regurgitant orifice (ERO) are most accurate provided there is not accompanying mitral regurgitation (MR). If both the aortic and mitral valves are regurgitant, planimetry of the aortic valve during transesophageal echocardiography (TEE) is the preferred method of determining valve area. As an indirect measure of the primary hemodynamic burden, the size and thickness of the LV generally reflect the dominant valve lesion. A dilated LV suggests AR; a normal sized LV with concentric hypertrophy implies AS (**149–154**, *Table 22*).

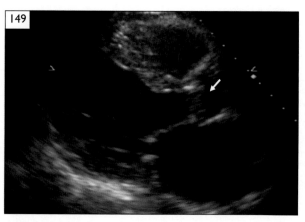

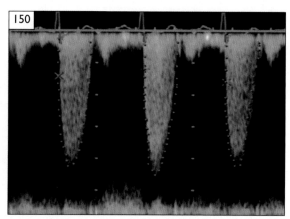

**149–154** Mixed aortic valve disease (aortic stenosis and aortic insufficiency) in an elderly patient. **149** Parasternal long axis echocardiographic view in systole demonstrating relatively fixed aortic valve cusps (arrow).
**150** Continuous wave Doppler interrogation of antegrade flow through the aortic valve. Both the peak velocity and the area under the traced velocity time curve (the velocity time integral) will be used to estimate valve area.

**151** Pulse wave Doppler interrogation of systolic flow through the left ventricular outflow tract. The area under this time velocity curve is the velocity time integral and will be used to estimate valve area using the continuity equation.

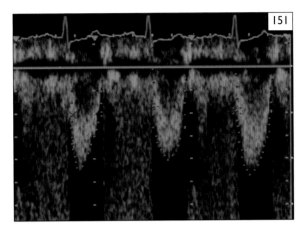

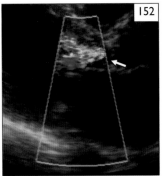

**152** Parasternal long axis view of same patient with Doppler color mapping of the regurgitant jet (arrow).

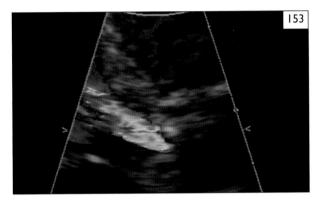

**153** Same image as (**152**) magnified to demonstrate more clearly the width of the regurgitant jet relative to the outflow tract. The ratio of the width of the jet to the width of the outflow tract is another means of characterizing the severity of aortic regurgitation.

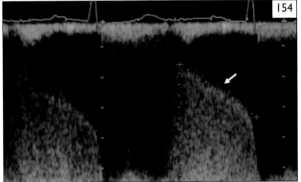

**154** Continuous wave Doppler interrogation of the regurgitant jet shown in **152** and **153**. The rate of decline in regurgitant flow velocity (the deceleration slope) is being measured (arrow) and will be used in the determination of pressure half-time. This is useful in characterizing the severity of aortic regurgitation. The diastolic timing is confirmed by the ECG tracing.

| **Table 22** Data table of hemodynamic and distance measurements used in calculation of valve area | | | | | | | |
|---|---|---|---|---|---|---|---|
| | **Measure used for calculation** | **Selected measure** | **1** | **2** | **3** | **4** | **5** |
| Ao $V_2$ max | 447 cm/sec | | 447 | | | | |
| Ao $V_2$ trace | 54.8 | | 54.8 | | | | |
| Ao $V_2$ VTI | 112 cm | | 112 | | | | |
| Ao dec slope | 400 cm/sec$^2$ | avg | 413 | 300 | 487 | | |
| AI max V | 449 cm/sec | avg | 447 | 432 | 469 | | |
| LV $V_1$ max | 87.2 cm/sec | avg | 83.3 | 88.2 | 81.9 | 95.2 | |
| LV $V_1$ trace | 2.14 | avg | 1.98 | 2.11 | 2.00 | 2.46 | |
| LV $V_1$ VTI | 24.0 cm | avg | 21.6 | 22.8 | 23.2 | 28.4 | |
| LVOT diam | 1.99 cm | avg | 1.89 | 2.09 | | | |
| Ao max PG | 79.8 mmHg (10.6 kPa) | Ao max PG2 | | | 76.7 mmHg (10.3 kPa) | | |
| Ao mean PG | 54.8 mmHg (7.3 kPa) | Ao mean PG2 | | | 52.7 mmHg (7.0 kPa) | | |
| Ao $P^1/_2$t | 329 msec | AVA(VD) | | | 0.605 cm$^2$ | | |
| AVA (ID) | 0.665 cm$^2$ | | | | | | |

AI: aortic insufficiency; Ao: aorta; AVA: aortic valve area; ID: integral-derived; LV: left ventricle; LVOT: left ventricle outflow tract; $P^1/_2$t: pressure half-time; PG: pressure gradient; V: velocity; VD: velocity-derived; VTI: velocity time integral.

## MANAGEMENT

Management of these patients is similar to that of single valve lesion patients, except that the threshold for surgery is lowered. Patients with severe AS with accompanying AR should be considered for surgery at larger estimated valve areas than patients with purely stenotic lesions. Patients with predominant AR but accompanying AS should be considered for surgery at smaller LV volumes than patients with purely regurgitant valves (Bonow *et al.*, 1998).

### Mitral stenosis and mitral regurgitation

#### ETIOLOGY

The underlying causes of mixed mitral valve disease are generally not different from those listed for mitral stenosis (MS) and mitral regurgitation (MR) listed in Chapters 7 and 9. One distinction is that LV dilatation and mitral annular distortion, which underlie many cases of functional MR, do not cause mixed disease. Left atrial (LA) or ventricular (LV) tumors may interfere with mitral valve function in both diastole and systole and hence cause mixed valve dysfunction. Another fairly unusual cause of mixed mitral disease is malfunction of a prosthetic valve.

#### PATHOPHYSIOLOGY

Mitral valves with elements of both obstruction and regurgitation place a volume load on the LV and a combined volume/pressure load on the LA. This favors the development of LA dilatation, atrial fibrillation and, if severe, LV dilatation.

#### CLINICAL PRESENTATION

The symptoms and signs of mixed MS/MR will develop earlier than would be expected in individual valve lesions of the same severity. In the echocardiography and catheterization laboratories, estimates of stenotic mitral valve area based on pressure gradients alone will be exaggerated by the additional transvalvular flow resulting from the MR. Doppler echocardiographic measurements may be the best method of determining the severity of MS in the presence of MR. In addition, measurements of pulmonary capillary wedge pressure (PCWP) or pulmonary artery systolic pressure during exercise may provide convincing evidence of the clinically important hemodynamic effect of seemingly moderate mixed mitral valve disease. A PCWP rising from normal to the upper 20s or 30s strongly supports cardiac dysfunction as the cause of dyspnea (Baim, 2000).

## MANAGEMENT

Similar to mixed aortic valve disease, clinical judgement is required in determining the appropriate time for surgical referral. In general, decision making will be more complex than with purely stenotic or regurgitant lesions. Intervention is often required before either of the component valve lesions reaches a severe grade. It is important to note that moderate MR is a contraindication to percutaneous balloon mitral valvuloplasty because of the risk of creating severe MR.

### References

Bonow RO, Carabello B, de Leon AC Jr, *et al.* (1998). ACC/AHA guidelines for the management of patients with valvular heart disease: a report of the American College of Cardiology/American Heart Association Task Force on practice guidelines (Committee on Management of Patients with Valvular Heart Disease). *Journal of the American College of Cardiology* 32:1486–1588.

Baim DS (2000). Exercise testing during cardiac catheterization. In: *Grossman's Cardiac Catheterization, Angiography and Intervention*, 6th edn. Lippincott ,Williams and Wilkins, Philadelphia, pp. 325–351.

# Chapter Sixteen

# Multiple Valve Disease

### Mitral stenosis/aortic stenosis

The most common cause of this combination is rheumatic heart disease. Pathophysiologically, it creates serial obstructions to flow. The left ventricle (LV) inflow obstruction prevents adequate LV filling and hence greatly reduces cardiac output. It must be recognized that because cardiac output is reduced, the aortic valve area (AVA) will be much lower than that suggested by the estimated transvalvular pressure gradient alone. It is, in effect, a form of 'low gradient' aortic stenosis (AS).

The presentation is characterized by symptoms of mitral stenosis (MS) and physical findings of AS. If suitable for valvotomy, percutaneous intervention of the mitral valve may be performed first, followed by consideration of aortic valve replacement (AVR) if the patient remains symptomatic (Bonow *et al.*, 1998). If surgery is necessary, every attempt should be made to repair, rather than replace, the mitral valve. AS in adults nearly always requires replacement (O'Rourke, 2001).

### Mitral stenosis/aortic regurgitation

This combination of valve lesions creates a particular challenge to physical diagnosis, since the MS minimizes the volume load on the LV, thereby blunting the characteristic exam findings of aortic regurgitation (AR). In addition, AR may further attenuate antegrade mitral valve flow by rapidly increasing LV diastolic pressure, and thereby decreasing the mitral transvalvular pressure gradient. As above, a sequential approach beginning with percutaneous mitral balloon valvuloplasty (PMBV) followed by consideration of AVR if symptoms persist, is a reasonable approach. Single valve replacement carries a lower morbidity and mortality risk than double valve surgery. In-hospital mortality for simultaneous mitral and aortic replacement is 5–10% in well-selected patients (O'Rourke, 2001).

### Mitral regurgitation/aortic stenosis

The increased afterload created by AS aggravates regurgitant flow through the mitral valve. In addition, because of the 'pressure relief valve' effect of mitral regurgitation (MR), LV systolic function may remain normal or hyperdynamic, and the transaortic pressure gradient will rarely rise excessively despite a critically stenosed aortic valve. Hence, AS aggravates MR, and MR obscures severe AS.

Clinically, this combination leads to increased pulmonary venous pressure, manifest by dyspnea and exercise intolerance out of proportion to the degree of individual valve disease. This is a common theme in patients suffering from multiple valve disease. Correct diagnosis requires careful consideration of clinical information and all laboratory data (**155–161**, *Table 23*).

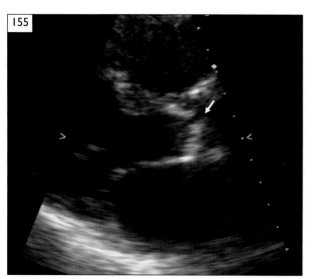

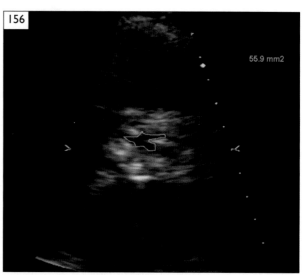

**155–161** Multiple valve disease (aortic stenosis and mitral regurgitation) in an 82-year-old female.
**155** Parasternal long axis echocardiographic view demonstrating the limited excursion of the aortic valve (arrow).
**156** Measurement of the aortic valve orifice area by planimetry in the parasternal short axis echocardiographic view.

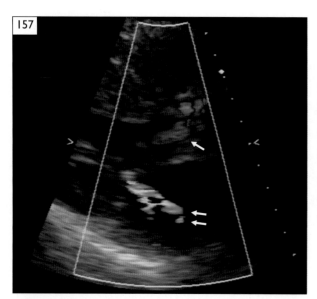

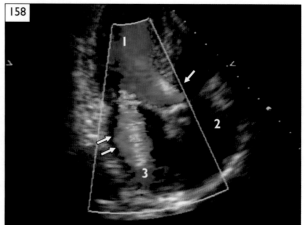

**158** Color flow map from the apical 3-chamber perspective demonstrating mitral regurgitation (double arrow) and high velocity antegrade flow in the left ventricular outflow tract (single arrow).
1: left ventricle; 2: ascending aorta; 3: left atrium.

**157** Parasternal long axis view with Doppler color flow mapping of the accompanying mitral regurgitation jet (double arrow) and antegrade flow in the left ventricular outflow tract (single arrow).

If both lesions are severe, AVR and mitral valve repair or replacement is indicated in the presence of symptoms, LV dysfunction, or pulmonary hypertension. However, in severe AS and moderate MR, relieving the LV outflow obstruction may significantly improve the MR by decreasing intraventricular pressure and, hence, reducing functional MR. Transesophageal echocardiography (TEE) and direct intraoperative inspection of the morphology of the mitral valve at the time of the AVR may clarify the need for simultaneous mitral valve replacement (MVR). If the mitral valve is anatomically normal, it is likely that repair or replacement is not necessary.

**159** Measurement of the width of the vena contracta as a semiquantitative measure of mitral regurgitation severity.

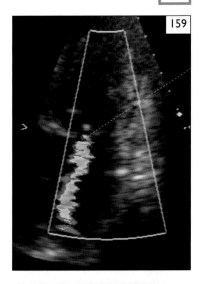

**160** Doppler color flow mapping of the mitral regurgitant jet demonstrating flow into the right upper pulmonary vein (arrow). 1: left ventricle; 2: right ventricle; 3: right atrium; 4: left atrium.

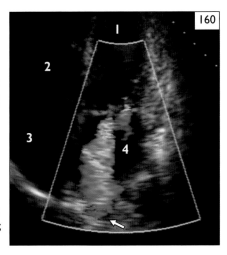

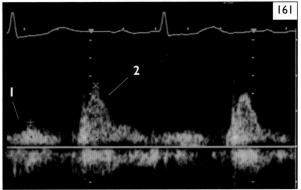

**161** Pulse wave Doppler assessment of flow in the right upper pulmonary vein. The blunting of systolic flow (1) relative to diastolic flow (2) is consistent with at least moderate mitral regurgitation (elevated left atrial pressure can also causes this).

**Table 23** Data table of hemodyanmic and distance measurements used in the continuity equation to determine an estimate of the aortic valve area

| | Measure used for calculation | Selected measure | 1 | 2 | 3 | 4 | 5 |
|---|---|---|---|---|---|---|---|
| Ao V$_2$ max | 285 cm/sec | avg | 277 | 269 | 253 | 295 | 333 |
| Ao V$_2$ trace | 20.0 | avg | 18.8 | 18.9 | 16.3 | 20.1 | 25.9 |
| AoV$_2$VTI | 63.5 cm | avg | 62.6 | 61.1 | 56.7 | 62.3 | 74.9 |
| LV V$_1$ max | 120 cm/sec | avg | 127 | 143 | 116 | 110 | 103 |
| LV V$_1$ trace | 3.36 | avg | 3.55 | 4.70 | 3.39 | 2.78 | 2.37 |
| LV V$_1$ VTI | 24.2 cm | avg | 26.3 | 29.2 | 24.7 | 23.9 | 17.3 |
| LVOT diam | 1.94 cm | | 1.94 | | | | |
| Ao max PG | 32.6 mmHg (4.4 kPa) | Ao max PG2 | | | 26.9 mmHg (3.6 kPa) | | |
| Ao mean PG | 20.0 mmHg (2.7 kPa) | Ao mean PG2 | | | 16.6 mmHg (2.2 kPa) | | |
| AVA (VD) | 1.24 cm$^2$ | AVA (ID) | | | 1.13cm$^2$ | | |

AVA: aortic valve area; Ao: aorta; ID: integral-derived; LV: left ventricle; LVOT: left ventricle outflow tract; PG: pressure gradient; V: velocity; VD: velocity-derived; VTI: velocity time integral.

In the situation of severe MR, the reduced forward stroke volume may create a situation of 'low gradient' AS. It can be difficult to determine whether the limited mobility of the aortic cusps is due to fixed stenosis or the low flow state (pseudostenosis). Some authorities advocate proceeding with AVR if the transaortic pressure gradient is >30 mmHg (4 kPa) (O'Rourke, 2001).

### Mitral regurgitation/aortic regurgitation

These valve lesions create additive volume loads on the LV. Therefore, the sequelae of dyspnea, LV dilatation, and systolic dysfunction appear sooner than anticipated based on consideration of either lesion alone. Doppler and 2D echocardiography provide much of the hemodynamic and anatomic data necessary for decisions regarding surgical timing.

### Prosthetic valves in multiple valve disease

Some investigators recommend double valve replacement over AVR and mitral valve repair, in light of retrospective evidence suggesting superior durability of the mitral prosthesis and comparable thromboembolic risk (Hamamoto et al., 2003).

Regarding the choice of valve prostheses, there appears to be little difference in thromboembolic and hemorrhagic complications of the newer bileaflet mechanical prostheses. Clinical investigators in British Columbia reported the results of 246 patients prospectively followed after undergoing multiple valve replacement surgery between 1989 and 1994 (Jamieson et al., 1998). Among these were 14 patients undergoing triple valve surgery. This study will be described in some detail to provide some measure of the approximate mortality and morbidity rates, as well as the importance of maintaining adequate anticoagulation. Nearly all received either a St. Jude or a CarboMedics bileaflet mechanical prosthesis. The international normalized ratio (INR) range recommended to patients and family physicians was 3.0–3.5.

Mean age was 57 years, 52.4% were in NYHA functional class II and 33.3% were in functional class IV. Mean follow-up was 2.42 ± 1.74 years. Early mortality was 12.2% (10% classified as valve-related, 40% nonvalvular cardiac causes, and 50% noncardiac and surgical causes). Risk factors for early mortality included class IV heart failure and advanced age. The late mortality rate was 3.85%/patient-year, with a valve-related rate of 2.2%/patient-year. The linearized rate of minor thromboembolic events was 2.52%/patient-year, while the rate of major thromboembolic events was 2.85%/patient-year (total of 5.4%/patient-year). Among the 31 patients experiencing thromboembolic events following discharge from the hospital, 76% were inadequately anticoagulated. Four patients experienced valve thrombosis requiring thrombolysis or emergent surgery. All four had inadequate anticoagulation. Valve prosthesis type (CarboMedics or St. Jude) was not a predictor of thromboembolic events or mortality. These finding underscore the importance of having a reliable process for tracking and ensuring proper anticoagulation based on the specific indication.

### References

Bonow RO, Carabello B, de Leon AC Jr, et al. (1998). ACC/AHA guidelines for the management of patients with valvular heart disease: a report of the American College of Cardiology/American Heart Association Task Force on Practice Guidelines (Committee on Management of Patients with Valvular Heart Disease). Journal of the American College of Cardiology 32:1486–1588.

Hamamoto M, Bando K, Kobayashi J, et al. (2003). Durability and outcome of aortic valve replacement with mitral valve repair versus double valve replacement. Annals of Thoracic Surgery 75(1):28–33.

Jamieson WRE, Munro AI, Miyagishima RT, et al. (1998). Multiple mechanical valve replacement surgery comparison of St. Jude Medical and CarboMedics prostheses. European Journal of Cardiothoracic Surgery 13(2):151–159.

O'Rourke RA (2001). Tricuspid valve, pulmonic valve, and multivalvular disease. In: Hurst's The Heart. V Fuster, RW Alexander, RA O'Rourke, et al. (eds). McGraw-Hill, New York, 1519–1531.

# Chapter Seventeen

# Infective Endocarditis

### Definition

Infection of the endocardium is a life-threatening illness. A delay in diagnosis may result in devastating embolic phenomena or dramatic cardiac decompensation. Its presentation, clinical course, treatment, and prognosis all vary with patient comorbidities, the specific pathogen, and the presence of prosthetic valves. While a detailed discussion is beyond the scope of this handbook, the main issues will be addressed.

### Etiology

The broad spectrum of organisms involved in infective endocarditis (IE) includes bacteria, fungi, mycobacterium, rickettsiae, chlamydia, and mycoplasma. However, the most prevalent infections are those of streptococci, staphylococci, enterococci, and Gram-negative coccobacilli (Karchmer, 2001) (**162**).

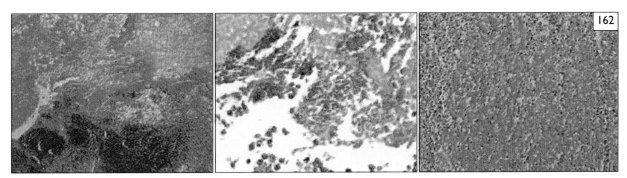

**162** Microscopic images at three different levels of magnification, demonstrating *Staphylococcus aureus* endocarditis. Note the plump Gram-positive cocci and the inflammatory response. (Courtesy of Nora Ratcliff, MD.)

## Pathophysiology

Endocarditis generally begins with damage to the endothelial lining of the heart, most commonly the valves, but any endothelial surface may be involved. Jets of abnormal blood flow are usually responsible for the endothelial damage, but any intravascular trauma may initiate the process. The combination of endothelial disruption and a hypercoagulable state produces foci of platelet and fibrin deposition. These foci constitute nonbacterial thrombotic endocarditis and serve as the milieu for bacterial attachment and proliferation (**163**).

The mitral valve, followed by the aortic valve, is most commonly affected. Characteristically, vegetations form on the downstream side of regurgitant flow (i.e. the atrial surface of mitral valves and the ventricular surface of aortic valves) (Patel and Steckelberg, 2000). Bacteria vary in their ability to attach and resist host defenses which explains, in part, the prevalence of the specific organisms mentioned earlier.

This seemingly superficial infection causes severe morbidity and mortality by several mechanisms including valve regurgitation via local tissue destruction (**164**), malfunction of prosthetic valves, elaboration of cytokines by activated leukocytes, embolic infarcts (**165**), hematogenous spread to distant organs via continuous bacteremia (**166**), and remote tissue damage from immune complex deposition (Karchmer, 2001).

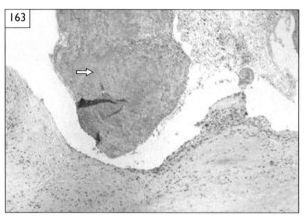

**163** Microscopic view of a murantic endocarditis lesion (arrow). Note the absence of bacteria and inflammatory cells. This consists primarily of thrombin and fibrin. (Courtesy of Nora Ratcliff, MD.)

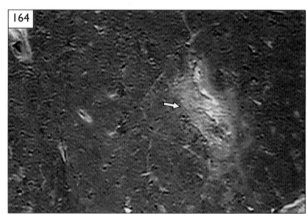

**164** Gross pathology specimen of a large vegetation attached to an aortic cusp (arrow). (Courtesy of Tom Farrell, MD.)

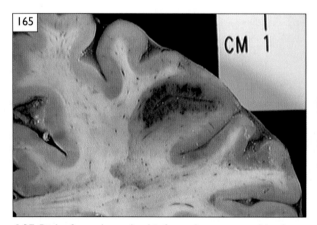

**165** Right frontal cerebral infarct that occurred in the context of nonbacterial thrombotic endocarditis and likely represents an embolic phenomenon. (Courtesy of Tom Farrell, MD.)

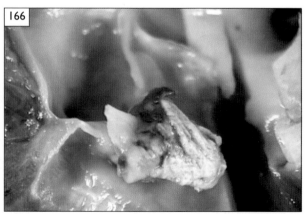

**166** Close up view of an embolic splenic abscess in a patient who died of *Staphylococcus aureus* endocarditis. (Courtesy of Tom Farrell, MD.)

## Clinical presentation

As one might expect from the variety of pathologic mechanisms, the clinical manifestations are diverse. They often include systemic symptoms (chills, sweats, anorexia, malaise, confusion) coupled with physical exam findings of fever and embolic phenomena (neurologic deficits, Roth's spots, Osler's nodes, petechiae, and Janeway lesions). A new or changing murmur is present in only 10–40% of patients. Splenomegaly and glomerulonephritis suggest immune complex disease.

Aerobic and anaerobic culture of three to six sets of blood specimens, each obtained 1 hour or more apart, is the most valuable diagnostic test. However, they may be negative in partially treated or culture-negative endocarditis. Transesophageal echocardiography (TEE) may confirm the diagnosis by demonstrating vegetations but cannot exclude the diagnosis (**167–170**). Care must be taken not to

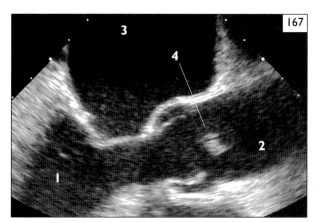

**167** Transesophageal view of a large vegetation attached to the undersurface of one of the aortic cusps. During diastole, the vegetation swung into the left ventricular outflow tract (1). 2: aorta; 3: left atrium; 4: vegetation. (Courtesy of Tim A. Beaver, MD.)

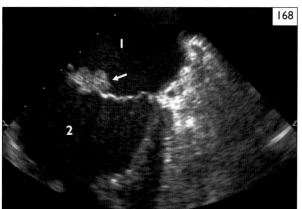

**168** Magnified echocardiography view of a large vegetation with a central echolucency consistent with abscess adherent to the atrial surface of the anterior mitral valve leaflet (arrow). 1; left atrium; 2: left ventricle.

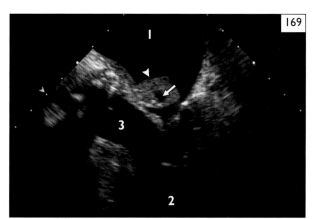

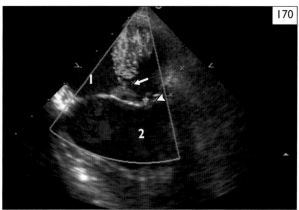

**169, 170** Mitral valve vegetation. **169** 2D transesophageal view of a large vegetation adherent to the mid portion of the anterior mitral leaflet (the A$_2$ segment). **170** Doppler color flow display suggesting the presence of a leaflet perforation. Note the flow through the perforation diverging above the vegetation (arrow) and the smaller jet of regurgitant flow through the leaflet coaptation site (arrowhead). 1: left atrium; 2: left ventricle; 3: left ventricle outflow.

mistake normal anatomic variations (e.g. Eustachian valves, nodules of Arantius, Lambl's excrescences) with vegetations (**171**). Both Von Reyn *et al.* (1981) and the Duke Endocarditis Service (Durack *et al.*, 1994) have published diagnostic criteria for IE. The Duke criteria incorporate echocardiographic findings (*Table 24*).

## Medical management
Prompt treatment with appropriate IV doses of antibiotics is essential to minimizing morbidity and mortality in these patients. The choice of antimicrobial agent depends on the etiologic organism, the nature of the infected valve (prosthetic or native),

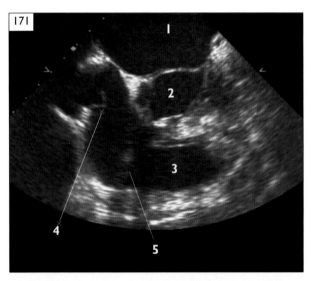

**171** A transesophageal view of a prominent Eustachian valve which lies at the junction of the inferior vena cava and the right atrium. This normal structure is sometimes mistaken for a vegetation of infective endocarditis. 1: left atrium; 2: aortic valve; 3: right ventricle; 4: Eustachian valve; 5: tricuspid valve.

---

**Table 24** Duke criteria for clinical diagnosis of infective endocarditis

**Major criteria**
Persistently positive blood cultures
    Typical organisms for endocarditis: *Streptococcus viridans*, *S. bovis*
    'HACEK' group, community-acquired *Staphylococcus aureus* or enterococci in the absence of primary focus
Persistent bacteremia: ≥2 positive cultures separated by ≥12 hours or ≥3 positive cultures ≥1 hour apart, or 70% blood culture samples positive if ≥4 are drawn

**Evidence of endocardial involvement**
    Positive echocardiogram
    Oscillating vegetation
    Abscesses
    Valve perforation
    New partial dehiscence of prosthetic valve
    New valvular regurgitation

**Minor criteria**
    Predisposing heart condition
    Mitral valve prolapse, bicuspid aortic valve, rheumatic or congenital heart disease, intravenous drug abuse

**Fever**
    Vascular phenomena
    Major arterial emboli, septic pulmonary emboli, mycotic aneurysm, intracranial hemorrhage, Janeway lesions

**Immunologic phenomena**
    Glomerulonephritis, Osler's nodes, Roth spots, rheumatoid factor
    Positive blood cultures: not meeting major criteria
    Echocardiogram: positive but not meeting major criteria

**Diagnosis**
    2 major criteria or
    1 major criterion plus 3 minor criteria or
    5 minor criteria

(Adapted from Bonow RO, Carabello B, de Leon AC Jr, et al. (1998). ACC/AHA guidelines for the management of patients with valvular heart disease. *Journal of the American College of Cardiology* **32**:1486–1588.)

and the immune status of the patient. The recommended duration of therapy ranges from 2 to 6 or more weeks (Bonow *et al.*, 1998). Current recommendations may be obtained from the American Heart Association on their website: www.americanheart.org (accessed 11/14/04).

## Surgical intervention

Excision of an infected valve and implantation of a prosthetic valve is recommended in the setting of severe congestive heart failure or cardiogenic shock, providing existing complications (e.g. severe central nervous system damage, multiorgan failure) do not preclude meaningful recovery (**172–174**). Less urgent

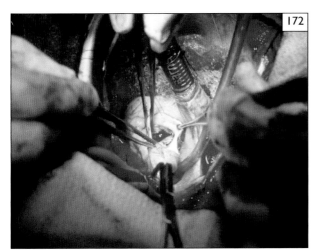

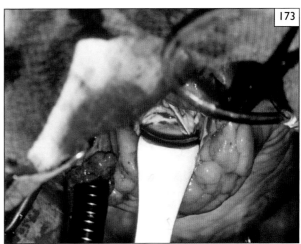

**172, 173** Intraoperative view of a patient with acute bacterial endocarditis involving the aortic valve. **172** Preserved valve architecture. **173** Vegetation adherent to the ventricular surface of the valve held in forcep. (Courtesy of John Sanders, MD.)

**174** Intraoperative photograph of a patient with endocarditis and vegetations adherent to the mitral valve. (Courtesy of John Sanders, MD.)

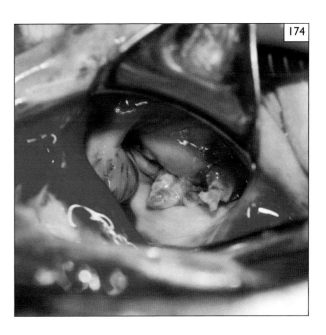

indications include perivalvular abscess, aneurysm formation, fever persisting beyond 7–10 days of appropriate antibiotics, fungal infection, prosthetic valve infection (175), and some cases of staphylococcal infection (Bonow *et al.*, 1998). The full AHA/ACC recommendations are outlined in *Tables 25, 26*.

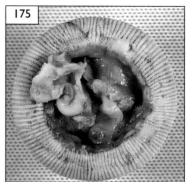

**175** This mitral bioprosthesis became infected and required resection. Note the prominent vegetations and the destruction of the valve leaflets. (Courtesy of Tom Farrell, MD.)

**Table 25** Recommendations for surgery for native valve endocarditis*

| Indication | Class |
| --- | --- |
| Acute AR or MR with heart failure | I |
| Acute AR with tachycardia and early closure of the mitral valve | I |
| Fungal endocarditis | I |
| Evidence of annular or aortic abscess, sinus, or aortic true or false aneurysm | I |
| Evidence of valve dysfunction and persistent infection after a prolonged period (7–10 days) of appropriate antibiotic therapy, as indicated by presence of fever, leukocytosis, and bacteremia, provided there are no noncardiac causes of infection | I |
| Recurrent emboli after appropriate antibiotic therapy | IIa |
| Infection with Gram-negative organisms or organisms with a poor response to antibiotics in patients with evidence of valve dysfunction | IIa |
| Mobile vegetations >10 mm | IIb |
| Early infections of the mitral valve that can likely be repaired | III |
| Persistent pyrexia and leukocytosis with negative blood cultures | III |

* Criteria also apply to repaired mitral and aortic allograft or autograft valves. Endocarditis defined by clinical criteria with or without laboratory verification; there must be evidence that function of a cardiac valve is impaired. AR: aortic regurgitation; MR: mitral regurgitation. (Adapted from Bonow RO, Carabello B, de Leon AC Jr, *et al.* (1998). ACC/AHA guidelines for the management of patients with valvular heart disease. *Journal of the American College of Cardiology* **32**:1486–1588.)

## Case study

A 43-year-old man was brought to the emergency room for evaluation of persistent sweats, chills, weight loss, and recent onset of confusion and drowsiness. His history was provided by one of his companions. Two months prior to admission he had left for Pakistan with a sponsored team of mountaineers to attempt a new climbing route on an 8000 m peak. Approximately 3 weeks prior to admission while fixing rope above camp III at 6500 m he started having mild fever and chills. He attributed this to fatigue and the effects of altitude, but when the symptoms continued at base camp he became a bit more concerned. Not wanting to jeopardize the expedition and his personal chance to reach the summit, he kept quiet and took ibuprofen on a scheduled basis. Despite this he became weaker and lost what little appetite he had. He gave up his rotation working high on the mountain. Several days later, a teammate discovered his sleeping bag soaked with sweat. Two fellow climbers accompanied him out of the mountains for the trek and long bus trip back to Islamabad, where he intended to fly home for medical care. He was having daily drenching sweats and had lost 9 kg (20 lb) since arriving in Pakistan. At the airport he felt somewhat short of breath at rest, but was able to board the plane without attracting attention. However, on the second

**Table 26** Recommendations for surgery for prosthetic valve endocarditis*

| Indication | Class |
|---|---|
| Early prosthetic valve endocarditis (first 2 months or less after surgery) | I |
| Heart failure with prosthetic valve dysfunction | I |
| Fungal endocarditis | I |
| Staphylococcal endocarditis not responding to antibiotic therapy | I |
| Evidence of paravalvular leak, annular or aortic abscess, sinus or aortic true or false aneurysm, fistula formation, or new-onset conduction disturbances | I |
| Infection with Gram-negative organisms or organisms with a poor response to antibiotics | I |
| Persistent bacteremia after a prolonged course (7–10 days) of appropriate antibiotic therapy with noncardiac causes of bacteremia | IIa |
| Recurrent peripheral embolus despite therapy | IIa |
| Vegetation of any size on or near the prosthesis | IIb |

*Criteria exclude repaired mitral valves or aortic allograft or autograft valves. Endocarditis is defined by clinical criteria with or without laboratory verification. (Adapted from Bonow RO, Carabello B, de Leon AC Jr, *et al.* (1998). ACC/AHA guidelines for the management of patients with valvular heart disease. *Journal of the American College of Cardiology* **32**:1486–1588.)

leg of the trip from Frankfurt to Chicago, he suffered the sudden onset of difficulty in speaking and right-sided weakness. The plane was diverted to Boston and the patient was taken from the airport to a large academic hospital.

His past history was remarkable for exceptional good health. He had never had any hospitalizations or operations. He took no medications. He was a lifelong nonsmoker and modest beer drinker (0–2 per day). His family history was unremarkable. Review of systems was remarkable for a dental abscess that had bothered him for a week about 1 month earlier. A team member had removed the tooth with multipurpose pliers he wore on his belt.

On exam he was a longhaired, unshaven, delirious man wearing dirty shorts and a T-shirt. His temperature was 39.2°C (102.5°F), blood pressure was 100/45 mmHg (13.3/6.0 kPa) in both arms, and his pulse rate was 98 bpm. He had splinter hemorrhages and Janeway lesions. His jugular venous pressure was below the level of the sternal angle and his carotid upstrokes were hyperdynamic. His chest exam revealed bibasilar crackles. His point of maximal intensity (PMI) was not displaced, but was hyperdynamic. He had no right ventricular lift. $S_1$ was normal, but was followed immediately by an ejection sound. $S_2$ was soft and there was a 2/6 decrescendo diastolic murmur heard along the left sternal border at held end-expiration while leaning forward. His spleen was enlarged. He had difficulty with word finding and mild right-sided weakness.

Urinalysis revealed red blood cell casts and bacteria. He had a leukocytosis, a normochromic, normocytic anemia, and an elevated platelet count. Three sets of blood cultures were collected 1 hour apart. An emergent computed tomography scan of the brain without contrast showed no evidence of intracranial hemorrhage. An urgent transthoracic echocardiogram revealed a hyperdynamic left ventricle with moderate aortic regurgitation (AR), and a vegetation adherent to the ventricular surface of the aortic valve.

He was admitted to the cardiac care unit and given fluids and intravenous antibiotics. The next morning a transesophageal echocardiogram confirmed the AR, the vegetation, but also revealed the presence of a complex echolucency at the base of the aortic valve, consistent with a valve abscess. Later that day the blood cultures grew *Streptococcus viridans*. After consultation with his family and friends, he was taken to the operating room and underwent resection of the aortic valve, debridement of all visible infection, and replacement with a bioprosthetic valve. Following the surgery he defervesced and his delirium cleared. Surveillance cultures grew nothing. He was discharged to a rehabilitation facility on his fourth hospital day, to complete his course of intravenous antibiotics and receive twice daily physical therapy. With this program he gained weight and strength steadily and by 2 weeks he was ambulating independently with the support of a cane. He had only mild word finding difficulties. Six months following discharge he was running 8 miles per day and was rock climbing. To his family's dismay, he was planning a winter climbing trip to Mexico.

COMMENTS

This vignette presents some of the common symptoms, findings, and natural history of infective endocarditis. Because of his remote location and disinterest in seeking prompt medical care he had developed advanced disease by the time of presentation. The presence of a valve abscess provided the indication for surgical valve replacement. The choice of a bioprosthetic valve was influenced by the patient's lifestyle that made warfarin therapy difficult, and by the notion that a bioprosthetic valve may be somewhat more resistant to infection.

## References

Bonow RO, Carabello B, de Leon AC Jr, *et al.* (1998). ACC/AHA guidelines for the management of patients with valvular heart disease: a report of the American College of Cardiology/American Heart Association Task Force on practice guidelines (Committee on Management of Patients with Valvular Heart Disease). *Journal of the American College of Cardiology* **32**:1486–1588.

Durack DT, Lukes AS, Bright DK (1994). New criteria for diagnosis of infective endocarditis: utilization of specific echocardiographic findings. Duke Endocarditis Service. *American Journal of Medicine* **96**:200–209.

Karchmer AW (2001). Infective endocarditis. In: *Heart Disease: A Textbook of Cardiovascular Medicine*. E Braunwald, DP Zipes, P Libby (eds). WB Saunders, Philadelphia, pp. 1723–1750.

Patel R, Steckelberg JM (2000). Infections of the heart. In: *Clinic Cardiology Review*, 2nd edn. JG Murphy (ed). Mayo. Lippincott, Williams' and Wilkins, Philadelphia, pp. 407–443.

Von Reyn CF, Levy BS, Arbeit RD, Friedland G, Crumpacker CS (1981). Infective endocarditis: an analysis based on strict case definitions. *Annals of Internal Medicine* **94**:505–518.

# Chapter Eighteen

# Drug-Induced Valvular Heart Disease

## Anorectic medication

### BACKGROUND

In light of the health risks of morbid obesity and the poor success rates of diet and exercise alone, there has been great interest in the pharmacologic therapy of obesity. Historically, pharmacologic doses of thyroid hormone and amphetamines have been employed. More recently, there have been a number of agents developed specifically to reduce appetite. One of the first was phentermine (Adipex – Gate Pharmaceuticals, Fastin – King Pharmaceuticals, Ionamin – Allscripts Healthcare Solutions), a nor-adrenergic central nervous system stimulant, approved by the Food and Drug Administration (FDA) in 1959 for use as an appetite suppressant. In 1973, fenfluramine (Pondimin – American Home Products Corporation), a sympathomimetic amine that promotes serotonin release and blocks its uptake, was approved for short-term use as a single agent in the treatment of obesity. Most recently, dexfenfluramine (Redux – Wyeth Ayres Pharmaceuticals), the dextroisomer of fenfluramine, was approved in 1996 as a single drug agent for obesity. Its activity is more specific for brain pathways than is fenfluramine.

Some investigators advocated the use of a combination of fenfluramine and phentermine, 'fen/phen', to suppress appetite by two separate mechanisms. In response to patient demand and some encouraging reports of efficacy with this combination therapy, approximately 18 million prescriptions were written for either fenfluramine or dexfenfluramine (Gaasch and Aurigemma, 2001).

### INITIAL REPORTS OF VALVULOPATHY

Suspicion of adverse valvular effects was first raised by investigators at the Mayo Clinic and MeritCare Medical Center in Fargo, North Dakota, US, who noticed valve lesions mimicking those of carcinoid syndrome (a condition of serotonin excess) and ergotamine use (Connolly et al., 1997). This initial report involved 24 women with an average age of 44 years taking the combination of fenfluramine (mean daily dose 60 mg) and phentermine (mean daily dose 30 mg) for 11 months (range 1–28). Curiously, the affected valves were both left- and right-sided, in contrast to the right-sided predominance seen in carcinoid syndrome. All valve lesions were regurgitant. Echocardiographically, the affected mitral valves (MV) were described as similar to those seen in patients with chronic rheumatic involvement, but lacking any evidence of obstruction. Typical findings included thickening and diastolic doming of the anterior leaflet. Thickening and shortening of the chordae tendineae with resultant tethering of the posterior mitral leaflet were common subvalvular findings. This combination of abnormalities frequently produced central regurgitation resulting from failure of leaflet coaptation (**176**). Affected aortic valves were thickened and retracted as well. When the tricuspid valve was involved, it too was thickened, with reduced mobility and evidence of diastolic doming and systolic malcoaptation. Eight of the 24 patients had Doppler echocardiographic or catheter based evidence of pulmonary hypertension (right ventricular systolic pressure 52–93 mmHg [6.9–12.4 kPa]). In the five patients who underwent valve surgery, the affected valves had a glistening white appearance (**177**). Histologically, the valves

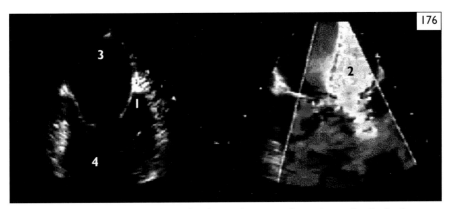

**176** Intraoperative transesophageal echocardiogram of a patient who had taken fenfluramine–phentermine. The image on the left shows a thickened mitral valve (1) during diastole. With the addition of color flow, the image on the right demonstrates severe mitral regurgitation (2) during systole. 3: left atrium; 4: left ventricle. (Reprinted from Connolly HM, Crary JL, McGoon MD *et al.* (1997). Valvular heart disease associated with fenfluramine-phentermine. *New England Journal of Medicine* **337**(9):581–588. With permission. Copyright Massachusetts Medical Society. All rights reserved.)

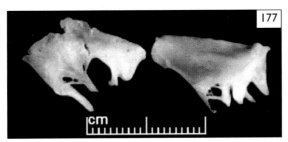

**177** Explanted mitral valve from a patient who had taken the anorectic drug combination fenfluramine–phentermine, demonstrating glistening white leaflets and chordae with mild-to-moderate irregular but diffuse thickening. (Reprinted from Connolly HM, Crary JL, McGoon MD, *et al.* (1997). Valvular heart disease associated with fenfluramine-phentermine. *New England Journal of Medicine* **337**(9):581–588. With permission. Copyright Massachusetts Medical Society. All rights reserved.)

were characterized by normal underlying valve architecture covered by 'stuck-on' plaques of proliferative myofibroblasts surrounded by extensive extracellular matrix (178–180). These features were described as 'identical to those seen in carcinoid or ergotamine-induced valve disease' (Connolly *et al.*, 1997).

Following a prepublication notification of this report, 28 additional case reports, all involving women, were received by the FDA and published as a letter in the same issue of the *New England Journal of Medicine* (Graham and Green, 1997). On the basis of these case reports, the manufacturer removed fenfluramine and dexfenfluramine from the market 1 month later, in September 1997. Subsequently, over 100 provider-initiated case reports were received by the FDA. All reports involved either fenfluramine or dexfenfluramine. None involved the noradrenergic agent phentermine used alone.

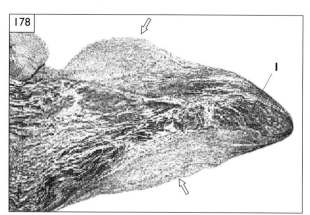

**178** Low power photomicrograph of a resected mitral valve from a patient who had taken fenfluramine–phentermine (elastic–van Gieson stain, ×36), displaying intact valve architecture with 'stuck-on' plaques (arrows). I: cord. (Reprinted from Connolly HM, Crary JL, McGoon MD, *et al.* (1997). Valvular heart disease associated with fenfluramine-phentermine. *New England Journal of Medicine* **337**(9):581–588. With permission. Copyright Massachusetts Medical Society. All rights reserved.)

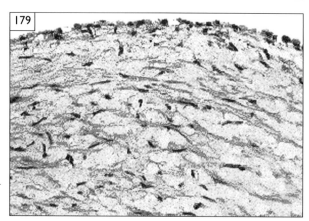

**179** A high-power view (hematoxylin and eosin, ×360) of the same valve shown in **178**, showing proliferative myofibroblasts in an abundant extracellular matrix. (Reprinted from Connolly HM, Crary JL, McGoon MD, *et al.* (1997). Valvular heart disease associated with fenfluramine-phentermine. *New England Journal of Medicine* **337**(9):581–588. With permission. Copyright Massachusetts Medical Society. All rights reserved.)

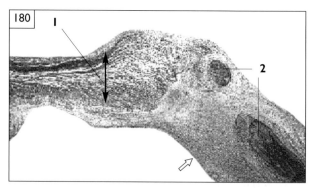

**180** A low-power view (Verhoeff–van Gieson stain, ×36) of a resected mitral valve from a female patient who had taken fenfluramine–phentermine. It shows an intact leaflet (1) and tendinous cord (2), with encasement by proliferative plaque (arrow). (Reprinted from Connolly HM, Crary JL, McGoon MD, *et al.* (1997). Valvular heart disease associated with fenfluramine-phentermine. *New England Journal of Medicine* **337**(9):581–588. With permission. Copyright Massachusetts Medical Society. All rights reserved.)

## SUBSEQUENT EPIDEMIOLOGIC STUDIES

A cross-sectional study published the next year compared the echocardiographic findings of 257 patients who had taken appetite suppressants in open label trials between 1994 and 1997 with the findings in 239 age-, sex-, height-, and body mass index-matched controls (Khan *et al.*, 1998). Using the case definition, defined by the FDA and the Center for Disease Control (CDC) as at least mild aortic regurgitation (AR) or at least moderate mitral regurgitation (MR), they reported a prevalence of 1.3% in controls, 12.8% in patients exposed to dexfenfluramine alone, 22.6% in those exposed to dexfenfluramine and phentermine in combination, and 25.2% in those exposed to fenfluramine and phentermine.

Prevalence figures reported by others have varied widely and therefore have introduced considerable uncertainty into the true impact of these drugs on valve disease. A cross-sectional study comparing 223 patients who took dexfenfluramine for a mean of 6.9 months to 189 controls, reported FDA/CDC-defined valve disease in 7.6% of the former and 2.1% of the latter (Shiveley *et al.*, 1999). The difference was driven primarily by an increase in mild AR (6.3% vs. 1.6%). The following year, another cross-sectional prevalence study (Gardin *et al.*, 2000) comparing 934 patients treated for at least 30 days with dexfenfluramine or fenfluramine–phentermine and 539 matched controls, reported a difference only in AR (8.9%, 13.7%, and 4.1% respectively). Still more data are available from a prospective, randomized trial of 366 patients assigned to immediate release dexfenfluramine, 352 assigned to sustained release dexfenfluramine, and 354 assigned to placebo for a mean duration of 72 days (Weissman *et al.*, 1998). Echocardiograms were performed at a median interval of 33 days after discontinuing the study medication. Using the FDA/CDC case definition, there was no statistical difference in the prevalence of regurgitant valve disease.

These negative findings may be attributable to the short duration of treatment. This is supported by the finding of a robust relationship between duration of therapy and prevalence of valve abnormalities in the Boston Collaborative Drug Surveillance Program, a population-based, nested case-control study of 6532 patients treated with dexfenfluramine, 2371 treated with fenfluramine, 862 treated with phentermine,

and 9281 untreated obese subjects (Jick *et al.*, 1998). The 5-year incidence per 10,000 persons was zero for those taking no medication or phentermine alone, 7.1 for those taking dexfenfluramine or fenfluramine for <4 months, and 35 per 10,000 for those taking the medications for ≥4 months.

## PATHOGENESIS

Because of the histologic similarity with carcinoid syndrome, a condition of serotonin excess, it is speculated that this neurotransmitter is responsible for the morphologic changes seen in **176–180**. Furthermore, serotonin is believed to stimulate fibroblast growth and fibrogenesis. However, there have been no reports linking some other medications which increase serotonin levels (e.g. fluoxetine, paroxetine, sertraline, buspirone) with valve plaque. This may be explained by receptor subtype specificity. A recent study examined radioligand binding of serotonin active drugs to eight different cloned human serotonin receptor subtypes (Rothman *et al.*, 2000). The investigators found that those drugs or their metabolites known or suspected to cause valvular lesions (ergotamine, methysergide, and fenfluramine) had preferentially high affinity for the 5-HT2B receptor subtype and were partial or full agonists. They concluded that 5-HT2B receptor activity is a necessary condition of drug toxicity.

## RECOMMENDATIONS

Although the relationship between these drugs and valve disease remains unclear, a legal settlement was reached between the manufacturers and plaintiffs who had used the medication. Prudent practice dictates that in light of the limited evidence available, fenfluramine and dexfenfluramine should be discontinued in anyone still taking the medication. Caution is advised in the use of any nonprescription anorectic drugs and supplements. Careful auscultation is advised in all exposed patients. If normal, it should be repeated in 6–8 months. Echocardiography is recommended in all patients with symptoms, murmurs, and in those whose body habitus precludes reliable detection of a murmur. Abnormal echocardiographic findings require follow-up with repeat study in 6–12 months, though current evidence suggests a low likelihood of progression (Weissman *et al.*, 2001). Bacterial endocarditis prophylaxis is recommended in patients with evidence of carcinoid-like valve disease. The recommendations from the US Department of Health and Human Services are listed in *Table 27*.

## Methysergide

Methysergide (Sansert – Novartis Pharmaceuticals) is an ergot derivative marketed for prophylaxis of vascular headache. Although it is a congener of ergotamine, it has somewhat different actions, with less vasoconstrictive properties, but significantly greater serotonin-like properties. Possibly as the result of 5-HT2B receptor activity mentioned above, it has been reported to cause fibrosis in a variety of locations including the retroperitoneum, lungs and pleura, penis (Peyronie's disease), and cardiac structures, including the aortic valve and MV (Misch, 1974; Redfield *et al.*, 1992). These lesions generally produce valvular regurgitation. In rare instances, fibrosis involves the aortic root, endocardium, or myocardium. To minimize the risk of this complication, it is recommended that the medication not be administered for >6 months continuously. A taper over 2–3 weeks, followed by a 'drug holiday' of 3–4 weeks is recommended. Patients taking this medication should be monitored for the development of murmurs and therapy should be discontinued if they develop. Patients with known valvular heart disease should not be prescribed this drug. With discontinuation of methysergide, regression of the valve lesions may occur.

## Ergotamine

Like methysergide, ergotamine (Cafergot – Novartis Pharmaceuticals, Ergomar – Harvest Pharmaceuticals, Wigraine – Organon) is an ergot derivative and is marketed for use in aborting or preventing vascular headaches. Its primary mechanism of action appears to be via partial agonist or antagonist activity against tryptaminergic, dopaminergic, and alpha-adrenergic receptors, varying with body site. It causes vasoconstriction of peripheral and cranial blood vessels and depression of central vasomotor centers. The predominant cardiovascular adverse effects derive from 'ergotism', excessive vasoconstriction presenting as cool extremities with greatly diminished pulses, hypertension, chest pain, electrocardiographic changes and, in severe cases, gangrene. However, pertinent to valvular cardiac disease, it has been associated with tissue fibrosis in a pattern similar to that of methysergide, with involvement of the retroperitoneum, pleura, and multiple heart valves (Wilke *et al.*, 1997). Affected valves resected at the time of valve replacement have demonstrated nodular thickening and fusion. On microscopy, proliferation of myofibroblasts with preservation of the underlying valve structure has been seen. The findings are very similar to those seen in carcinoid heart disease, methysergide toxicity, and fenfluramine/dexfenfluramine heart disease described above (Hendrikx *et al.*, 1996). Ergotamine appears less likely to cause fibrosis than methysergide, which has greater tryptaminergic activity.

**Table 27** Recommendations for management of patients who have used anorectic drugs*

| Indication | Class |
| --- | --- |
| Discontinuation of the anorectic drug(s) | I |
| Cardiac physical examination | I |
| Echocardiography in patients with symptoms, heart murmurs, or associated physical findings | I |
| Doppler echocardiography in patients for whom cardiac auscultation cannot be performed adequately because of body habitus | I |
| Repeat physical examination in 6–8 months for those without murmurs | IIa |
| Echocardiography in all patients before dental procedures in the absence of symptoms, heart murmurs, or associated physical findings | IIb |
| Echocardiography in all patients without heart murmurs | III |

* Fenfluramine or dexfenfluramine or the combination of fenfluramine–phentermine or dexfenfluramine–phentermine. (Adapted from Bonow RO, Carabello B, de Leon AC Jr, et al. (1998). ACC/AHA guidelines for the management of patients with valvular heart disease. *Journal of the American College of Cardiology* **32**:1486–1588.)

## Pergolide

Pergolide (Permax – Amarin) is an ergot-derived dopaminergic receptor agonist, used in the treatment of Parkinson disease and restless leg syndrome. Beginning in the mid-1990s, reports were published associating pergolide with pericardial, retroperitoneal, and pleural fibrosis. Recently, a case series of three patients with severe, unexplained tricuspid regurgitation (**181**, **182**) was published (Pritchett *et al.*, 2002). Two of the patients required valve replacement surgery; one, tricuspid valve replacement alone, the other, replacement of the aortic, mitral, and tricuspid valves. Grossly, the resected valves and subvalvular apparatus appeared thickened. Histologically, the valves all displayed plaques of fibroendocardial thickening with preservation of the underlying valvular architecture, mimicking the changes seen in carcinoid heart disease, methysergide, ergotamine, and fenfluramine use (**183**, **184**). None of the patients had biochemical evidence of carcinoid syndrome or a history of use of these drugs.

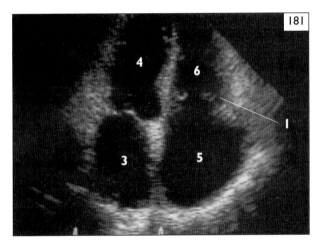
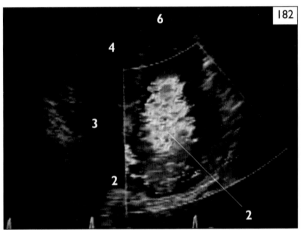

**181, 182** Tricuspid valve thickening. **181** Apical 4-chamber view of transthoracic echocardiogram during systole showing tricuspid valve leaflet thickening and retraction (1). **182** The resulting leaflet malcoaptation during systole results in severe tricuspid valve regurgitation (2) as seen on a color flow Doppler image. 3: left atrium; 4: left ventricle; 5: right atrium; 6: right ventricle. (From Pritchett AM, Morrison JF, Edwards WD, Schaff HV, Connolly HM, Espinosa RE (2002). Valvular heart disease in patients taking pergolide. *Mayo Clinic Proceedings* **77**(12):1280–1286. With permission.)

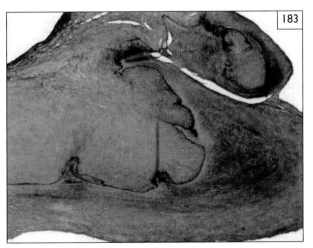
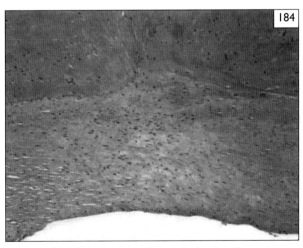

**183, 184** Photomicrographs of surgically resected tricuspid valve. **183** Fibroelastic proliferative lesion along the ventricular surface of the distal aspect of the leaflet, with encasement of the tendinous cord (Verhoeff–van Gieson, ×40). **184** Interface between the intact leaflet (above) and proliferative lesion (below) (hematoxylin and eosin, ×100). (From Pritchett AM, Morrison JF, Edwards WD, Schaff HV, Connolly HM, Espinosa RE (2002). Valvular heart disease in patients taking pergolide. *Mayo Clinic Proceedings* **77**(12):1280–1286. With permission.)

## References

Connolly HM, Crary JL, McGoon MD, et al. (1997). Valvular heart disease associated with fenfluramine-phentermine. *New England Journal of Medicine* **337**(9):581–588.

Gaasch WH, Aurigemma GP (2001). Valvular heart disease induced by anorectic drugs. Up To Date (version 11.1) available on the world wide web at www.uptodate.com (03/12/03).

Gardin JM, Schumacher D, Constantine G, et al. (2000). Valvular abnormalities and cardiovascular status following exposure to dexfenfluramine or phentermine/fenfluramine. *Journal of the American Medical Association* **283**:1703–1709.

Graham DJ, Green L (1997). Further cases of valvular heart disease associated with fenfluramine- phentermine [letter]. *New England Journal of Medicine* **337**(9):635.

Hendrikx M, Van Dorpe J, Flameng W, Daenen W (1996). Aortic and mitral valve disease induced by ergotamine therapy for migraine: a case report and review of the literature. *Journal of Heart Valve Disease* **5**(2):235–237.

Jick H, Visilakis C, Weinrauch LA, Meier CR, Jick SS, Derby LE (1998). A population-based study of appetite-suppressant drugs and the risk of cardiac-valve regurgitation. *New England Journal of Medicine* **339**:719–724.

Khan MA, Herzog CA, St. Peter JV, et al. (1998). The prevalence of cardiac valvular insufficiency assessed by transthoracic echocardiography in obese patients treated with appetite-suppressant drugs. *New England Journal of Medicine* **339**:713–718.

Misch KA (1974). Development of heart valve lesions during methysergide therapy. *British Medical Journal* **2**(915):365–366.

Pritchett AM, Morrison JF, Edwards WD, Schaff HV, Connolly HM, Espinosa RE (2002). Valvular heart disease in patients taking pergolide. *Mayo Clinic Proceedings* **77**(12):1280–1286.

Redfield MM, Nicholson WJ, Edwards WD, Tajik AJ (1992). Valve disease associated with ergot alkaloid use: echocardiographic and pathologic correlations. *Annals of Internal Medicine* **117**(1):50–52.

Rothman RB, Baumann MH, Savage JE, et al. (2000). Evidence for possible involvement of 5-HT 2B receptors in the cardiac valvulopathy associated with fenfluramine and other serotonergic medications. *Circulation* **102**:2836–2841.

Shively BK, Roldan CA, Gill EA, et al. (1999). Prevalence and determinants of valvulopathy in patients treated with dexfenfluramine. *Circulation* **100**:2161–2167.

Weissman NJ, Tighe JF, Gottdiener JS, Gwynne JT, for the Sustained Release Dexfenfluramine Study Group (1998). An assessment of heart valve abnormalities in obese patients taking dexfenfluramine, sustained dexfenfluramine, or placebo. *New England Journal of Medicine* **339**:725–732.

Weissman NJ, Panza JA, Tighe JF, Gwynne JT (2001). Natural history of valvular regurgitation 1 year after discontinuation of dexfenfluramine therapy. A randomized, double-blind, placebo-controlled trial. *Annals of Internal Medicine* **134**:267–273.

Wilke A, Hesse H, Hufnagel G, Maisch B (1997). Mitral, aortic, and tricuspid valvular heart disease associated with ergotamine therapy for migraine. *European Heart Journal* **18**(4):701.

# Chapter Nineteen

# Prosthetic Heart Valves

### Types of prosthetic valves

Prosthetic heart valves were first implanted in humans in 1960. Valves made entirely of manufactured materials are known as mechanical valves, while those containing animal tissue (porcine or bovine) or preserved human tissue (homografts) are called bioprostheses.

Mechanical valves follow one of two main designs: ball and cage or tilting disk. Tilting disk valves may be single disk or bileaflet in form. While the greatest cumulative experience resides with the Starr–Edwards ball and cage valve, the mechanical valve most frequently implanted today is the St. Jude bileaflet tilting disk valve. Its popularity is due in large part to its low flow resistance relative to other mechanical designs. In the interest of minimizing thrombogenicity, all tilting disk valves have some 'built-in' regurgitation designed to 'wash off' the valve surface at the onset of each diastole (185). This built-in regurgitation must be distinguished from abnormal perivalvular regurgitation (186).

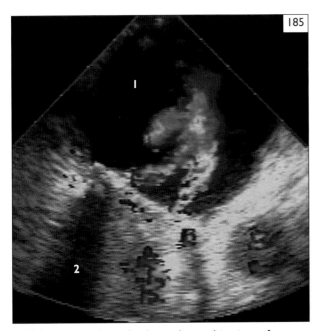

**185** A transesophageal echocardiographic view of a bileaflet tilting disc prosthesis in the mitral position during early diastole. Note the three distinct regurgitant jets which serve to 'wash off' the surface of the mechanical leaflets. 1: left atrium; 2: left ventricle. (Courtesy of Timothy A. Beaver, MD.)

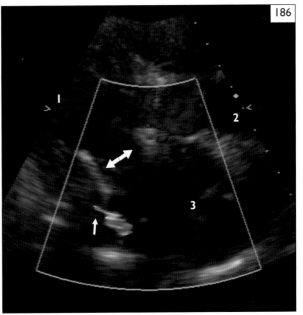

**186** Echocardiography of a perivalvular leak. A 'zoomed in' view from the parasternal long axis perspective of a patient with a prosthetic mitral valve (double headed arrow) and a posteriorly located small perivalvular leak (single headed arrow). 1: left ventricle; 2: ascending aorta; 3: left atrium.

The animal valves are meticulously hand sewn on a frame, a technique which requires years to master. They are designed to have no regurgitation. An important design feature for both mechanical and tissue prostheses in the mitral position is the profile (i.e. the degree to which it extends into the ventricle from the valve plane). A high profile valve angulated towards the left ventricular outflow tract may cause obstruction (**187, 188**).

### Selection of valve prosthesis

Mechanical valves generally offer greater durability in positions of high hemodynamic stress (i.e. the aortic position) and offer the predictability and quality control of manufactured materials. However, they are thrombogenic and require strict maintenance of moderate to high levels of anticoagulation (international normalized ratio 2.5–3.5), with the attendant risk and inconvenience.

Bioprostheses are rendered antigen free by glutaraldehyde fixation. Therefore, they require no immunosupression and no antithrombotic therapy. However, their limited durability in comparison to mechanical prostheses may mandate repeat valve surgery when the patient is older and frailer. The newer bovine pericardial bioprostheses may be more durable than porcine valves. In a study of 292 bovine valves in the aortic position followed for a mean of 7.8 years, the 10-year actuarial freedom from structural deterioration was 91.2% (Cosgrove *et al.*, 1995).

As a rough guideline, mechanical prostheses offer better survival in patients <65 years old undergoing aortic valve replacement and patients <50 years old undergoing mitral valve repair. Older patients and

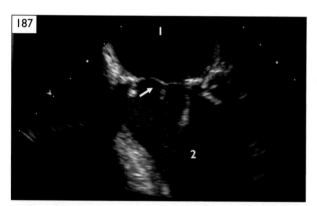

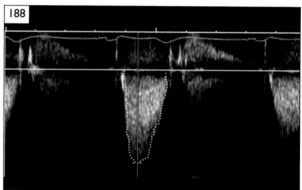

**187, 188** Transesophageal echocardiography of a patient with a prosthetic mitral valve which partially obstructs the left ventricular outflow tract. **187** 2D view of the prosthetic mitral valve (arrow). Note the angulation of the valve towards the outflow tract. 1: left atrium; 2: left ventricle. **188** Apical continuous wave Doppler interrogation through the left ventricular outflow tract and aortic valve, demonstrating an increased peak velocity (3 m/s) related to the prosthetic mitral valve. 1: left atrium; 2: left ventricle.

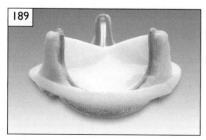

**189** Carpentier–Edwards Perimount pericardial bioprosthesis for the aortic position. (Copyright Edwards Lifesciences LLC, printed with permission.)

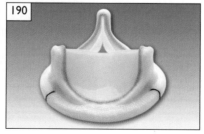

**190** Carpentier–Edwards Perimount pericardial bioprosthesis for the mitral position. (Copyright Edwards Lifesciences LLC, printed with permission.)

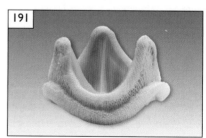

**191** Carpentier–Edwards SAV bioprosthesis for the aortic position. (Copyright Edwards Lifesciences LLC, printed with permission.)

those at greatly increased risk from anticoagulation may be better served with a bioprosthesis (Bonow *et al.*, 1998). An independent need for anticoagulation (e.g. atrial fibrillation) favors the use of a mechanical valve regardless of age. Ultimately, unique features of each patient must be considered in the selection of prosthetic valves. Food and Drug Administration approved prosthetic heart valves are listed in *Table 28*. Examples of the more commonly used bioprosthetic valves are shown in **189–194**. A variety

| **Table 28** FDA-approved prosthetic heart valves | | |
|---|---|---|
| **Company** | **Device name** | **Date approved** |
| Alliance Medical Technologies Inc. | Monostrut cardiac valve prosthesis | 1997 |
| ATS Medical Centre | ATS open pivot bileaflet heart valve | 2000 |
| Baxter Healthcare Corp. | Starr–Edwards silastic ball heart valve prosthesis | 1991 |
| Carbomedics Inc. | Carbomedics prosthetic heart valve | 1993 |
| Cutter Laboratories Inc. | Heart valve prosthetic cooley-cutter | 1977 |
| Edwards Lifesciences LLC | Carpentier–Edwards Perimount plus pericardial bioprosthesis | 2000 |
| Edwards Lifesciences LLC | Edwards Prima Plus stentless bioprosthesis model 2500P | 2001 |
| Edwards Lifesciences LLC | Carpentier–Edwards SAV bioprosthesis model 2650 (aortic) | 2002 |
| Edwards Lifesciences LLC | Carpentier–Edwards Perimount magna pericardial bioprosthesis model 3000 aortic | 2003 |
| Edwards Lifesciences LLC | Carpentier–Edwards Perimount pericardial bioprosthesis | 2001 |
| Medical Carbon Research Instit. LLC | On-X® prosthetic heart valve model ONXA | 2001 |
| Medical Inc. | Omniscience prosthetic cardiac valve | 1988 |
| Medtronic Inc. | Medtronic Hall prosthetic heart valve/Hall easy fit | 2003 |
| Medtronic Inc. | Medtronic mosaic porcine bioprosthetic heart valve | 2000 |
| Medtronic Inc. | Hall® easy-fit prosthetic heart valve | 2001 |
| Medtronic Inc. | Medtronic Hall® prosthetic heart valve | 1982 |
| Medtronic Inc. | Hancock II porcine bioprosthesis | 1999 |
| Medtronic Inc. | Medtronic freestyle aortic root bioprosthesis | 1997 |
| St. Jude Medical Inc. | St. Jude Medical regent mechanical heart valve (aortic) | 2002 |
| St. Jude Medical Inc. | Toronto SPV valve | 1997 |

FDA: Food and Drug Administration. (Table adapted from FDA website, April 2004.)

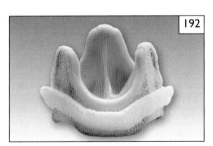

**192** Carpentier–Edwards SAV bioprosthesis for the mitral position. (Copyright Edwards Lifesciences LLC, printed with permission.)

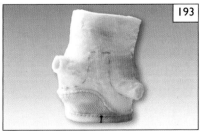

**193** Edwards Prima Plus® stentless bioprosthesis for the aortic position. (Copyright Edwards Lifesciences LLC, printed with permission.)

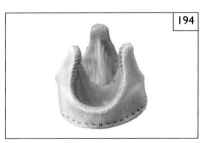

**194** St. Jude Toronto stentless prosthetic valve. (Copyright St. Jude Medical Inc. 2004. This image is provided courtesy of St. Jude Medical Inc. All rights reserved.)

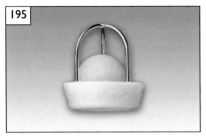

**195** Starr–Edwards silastic ball valve for the aortic position. (Copyright Edwards Lifesciences LLC, printed with permission.)

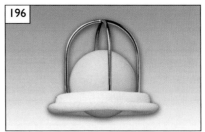

**196** Starr–Edwards silastic ball valve for the mitral position. (Copyright Edwards Lifesciences LLC, printed with permission.)

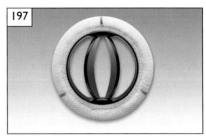

**197** Edwards MIRA™ ultra finesse (only available outside the USA). (Copyright Edwards Lifesciences LLC, printed with permission.)

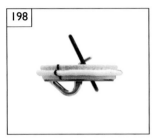

**198** Medtronic Hall single tilting disk prosthesis seen from the side. (Copyright Medtronics Inc., printed with permission.)

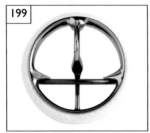

**199** Medtronic Hall single tilting disk prosthesis seen from above. (Copyright Medtronics Inc., printed with permission.)

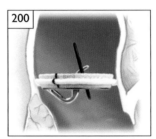

**200** Schematic diagram of Medtronic Hall single tilting disk prosthesis in the aortic root. (Copyright Medtronics Inc., printed with permission.)

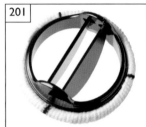

**201** SJM regent valve, a bileaflet tilting valve. (Copyright St. Jude Medical, Inc. 2004. This image is provided courtesy of St. Jude Medical, Inc. All rights reserved.)

**Table 29** Antithrombotic therapy with prosthetic heart valves

| | Warfarin (INR 2.0–3.0) | Warfarin (INR 2.5–3.5) | Aspirin (80–100 mg) |
|---|---|---|---|
| **Mechanical prosthetic valves** | | | |
| First 3 months after replacement | | + | + |
| After first 3 months | | | |
| Aortic valve[†] | + | | + |
| Aortic valve + 'risk factor'* | | + | + |
| Mitral valve | | + | + |
| Mitral valve + 'risk factor'* | | + | + |
| **Biological prosthetic valves** | | | |
| First 3 months after replacement | | + | + |
| After first 3 months | | | |
| Aortic valve | | | + |
| Aortic valve + 'risk factor'* | + | | + |
| Mitral valve | | | + |
| Mitral valve + 'risk factor'* | | + | + |

Note: Depending on patient's clinical status, antithrombotic therapy must be individualized. * Risk factors: atrial fibrillation, left ventricular dysfunction, previous thromboembolism, and hypercoagulable condition. [†]INR should be maintained between 2.5 and 3.5 for aortic disk valves and Starr–Edwards valves. INR: international normalized ratio. (Adapted from McAnulty JH and Rahimtoola SH (1998). Antithrombotic therapy in valvular heart disease. In: *Hurst's The Heart, Arteries, and Veins*, 9th edn. R Schlant, RW Alexander (eds). McGraw–Hill Publishing Co, New York, pp. 1867–1874.)

of popular mechanical prostheses are shown in **195–201**.

The ACC/AHA guideline regarding antithrombotic therapy with prosthetic valves based on recommendations from McAnulty and Rahimtoola (1998) is shown in *Table 29*. Perioperative (noncardiac surgery) management of antithrombotic therapy is outlined in *Table 30*. Recommendations regarding follow-up of patients with prosthetic valves is shown in *Table 31*.

---

**Table 30** Antithrombotic therapy in patients requiring noncardiac surgery dental care

**Usual approach**

| | |
|---|---|
| If patient on warfarin | Stop 72 hours before procedure<br>Restart in the afternoon on the day of procedure, or after control of active bleeding |
| If patient on aspirin | Stop 1 week before procedure<br>Restart the day after procedure or after control of active bleeding |

**Unusual circumstances**

| | |
|---|---|
| Very high risk of thrombosis if off warfarin* | Stop warfarin 72 hours before procedure<br>Start heparin when INR falls below 2.0†<br>Stop heparin 6 hours before procedure<br>Restart heparin within 24 hours of procedure and continue until warfarin can be restarted and INR=2.0 |
| Surgery complicated by postoperative bleeding | Start heparin as soon after surgery as deemed safe and maintain PTT at 55–70 seconds until warfarin restarted and INR =2.0 |
| Very low risk from bleeding‡ | Continue antithrombotic therapy |

* Clinical judgement: consider this approach if recent thromboembolus, Björk–Shiley valve, or three 'risk factors' are present. Risk factors are atrial fibrillation, left ventricular dysfunction, previous thromboembolism, hypercoagulable condition, and mechanical prosthesis. One risk factor is sufficient to consider heparin in patients with mechanical valves in mitral position. †Heparin can be given in the outpatient setting before and after surgery. ‡For example, local skin surgery, teeth cleaning, and treatment for caries. INR: international normalized ratio; PTT: partial thromboplastin time. (Adapted from Bonow RO, Carabello B, de Leon AC Jr, et al. (1998). ACC/AHA guidelines for the management of patients with valvular heart disease. *Journal of the American College of Cardiology* **32**:1486–1588.)

---

**Table 31** Recommendations for follow-up strategy of patients with prosthetic heart valves

| Indication | Class |
|---|---|
| History, physical exam, ECG, chest X-ray, echocardiogram, complete blood count, serum chemistries, and INR (if indicated) at first postoperative outpatient evaluation* | I |
| Radionuclide angiography or magnetic resonance imaging to assess LV function if result of echocardiography is unsatisfactory | I |
| Routine follow-up visits at yearly intervals with earlier reevaluations for change in clinical status | I |
| Routine serial echocardiograms at time of annual follow-up visit in absence of change in clinical status | IIb |
| Routine serial fluoroscopy | III |

*This evaluation should be performed 3–4 weeks after hospital discharge. In some settings, the outpatient echocardiogram may be difficult to obtain; if so, an inpatient echocardiogram may be obtained before hospital discharge. ECG: electrocardiogram; INR: international normalized ratio; LV: left ventricular. (Adapted from Bonow RO, Carabello B, de Leon AC Jr, et al. (1998). ACC/AHA guidelines for the management of patients with valvular heart disease. *Journal of the American College of Cardiology* **32**:1486–1588.)

## References

Bonow RO, Carabello B, de Leon AC Jr, *et al.* (1998). ACC/AHA guidelines for the management of patients with valvular heart disease: a report of the American College of Cardiology/American Heart Association Task Force on Practice Guidelines (Committee on Management of Patients with Valvular Heart Disease). *Journal of the American College of Cardiology* **32**:1486–1588.

Cosgrove DM, Lytle BW, Taylor PC, *et al.* (1995). The Carpentier–Edwards pericardial aortic valve: ten-year results. *Journal of Thoracic and Cardiovascular Surgery* **110**:651–662.

McAnulty JH, Rahimtoola SH (1998). Antithrombotic therapy in valvular heart disease. In: *Hurst's The Heart, Arteries, and Veins*, 9th edn. R Schlant, RW Alexander (eds). McGraw-Hill Publishing Co, New York, pp. 1867–1874.

# Chapter Twenty

# Pregnancy and Valvular Heart Disease

**Pregnancy in women without valvular heart disease**

PHYSIOLOGY

One of the most striking cardiovascular adaptations to pregnancy is the expansion in total blood volume of approximately 50%. Since plasma volume increases more than red blood cell mass (30–50% vs. 20–30%), a mild anemia normally develops. Accompanying this is a steady increase in cardiac output which reaches its maximum between 20 and 33 weeks of gestation. This rise in cardiac output results primarily from an increase in stroke volume, and secondarily from an increase in heart rate. The uterine circulation and endocrine effects result in a decrease in systemic vascular resistance (SVR) which, in turn, facilitates the increase in stroke volume. Oxygen consumption increases by approximately 30% during pregnancy. This increase is shared by the mother and fetus, with the uterus itself claiming up to 18% of total oxygen consumption.

In the later stages of pregnancy, the weight of the fetus and the uterus may dramatically influence cardiovascular performance. In the supine position, they may compress the inferior vena cava and reduce systemic venous return and, therefore, cardiac output. The left lateral decubitus position minimizes compression of the inferior vena cava. During labor and delivery, cardiac output increases further in the context of pain, anxiety, and physical exertion. Uterine contractions are often accompanied by increases in diastolic and systolic blood pressure. Following delivery, a surge in preload is produced by the redistribution of uterine blood into the systemic circulation and by the relief of partial caval obstruction.

Other changes relevant to the cardiovascular system include a relative hypercoaguable state stemming from a decrease in protein S activity, lower extremity venous hypertension, and blood stasis. Vessel wall strength may be impaired by both the inhibition of collagen deposition by estrogen and by an increase in circulating elastases.

PHYSICAL EXAM

Consistent with the increase in cardiac output and diminished SVR noted above, the skin over the extremities of pregnant women is typically warm. Peripheral edema is common. The peripheral pulses are mildly hyperdynamic, and the jugular venous pressure is mildly increased with prominent a and v pulsations. The thyroid gland may be mildly enlarged and diaphragmatic excursion diminished. Precordial palpation usually reveals an enlarged and laterally displaced apical impulse. $S_1$ is often loud with prominent physiologic splitting. $S_2$ is usually physiologically split and may widen and become persistently split late in pregnancy. An $S_3$ is heard in 80% of pregnant women. Similarly, an early peaking systolic ejection murmur arising from the pulmonary outflow tract is heard in over 90% of women. Diastolic murmurs are much less common, occurring in only 18% of normal pregnant women. A continuous murmur may be heard. Common sources include a cervical venous hum (confirmed by compression of the ipsilateral jugular vein) or a mammary soufflé which arises from the hyperemia associated with engorged breasts (confirmed by obliteration of the murmur by firm pressure on the diaphragm of the stethoscope). An $S_4$, a murmur louder than grade II/VI, a diastolic murmur, and fixed splitting of the second heart sound are uncommon and should prompt further investigations.

ECHOCARDIOGRAPHY

Along with the increase in total circulating blood volume, normal findings in pregnancy include mild ventricular dilatation and mild right-sided (tricuspid and pulmonic) valve regurgitation. Mild annular dilatation may also produce some mild mitral regurgitation.

## Maternal and fetal outcomes in valvular heart disease

Data on the outcomes of pregnancy in valvular heart disease (VHD) are limited. One study from the University of Southern California School of Medicine (Hameed *et al.*, 2001) retrospectively evaluated 66

pregnancies in 64 women with VHD and compared them to 66 women without VHD matched for age, ethnicity, obstetrical and medical history, time of initial prenatal care, and year of pregnancy. The investigators focused on stenotic valve lesions involving the aortic, mitral, and pulmonic valves and excluded patients with prosthetic valves. Patients were stratified into mild, moderate, and severe stenosis based on estimated valve area. Fifty-five percent were in New York Heart Association (NYHA) heart failure functional class I, 42% in class II, and 3% in class III. Maternal clinical outcomes included mortality, change in NYHA functional class, incidence of new congestive heart failure

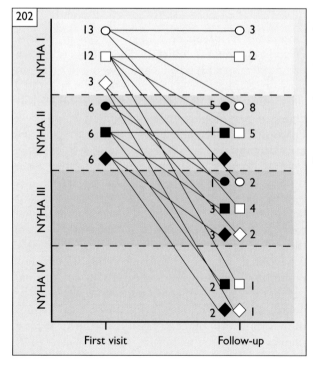

**202** Change in New York Heart Association (NYHA) functional class between first visit and follow-up during pregnancy in patients with predominant mitral valve disease. Circles: mild mitral stenosis; squares: moderate mitral stenosis; diamonds: severe mitral stenosis. Open symbols: NYHA functional class I on presentation; closed symbols: NYHA functional class II on presentation. (Adapted from Hameed A, Karaalp IS, Tummala PP, *et al.* (2001). The effect of valvular heart disease on maternal and fetal outcome of pregnancy. *Journal of the American College of Cardiology* **37**:893–899.)

(CHF), nonobstetric hospitalizations, new or worsening arrhythmias, need to start or increase cardiac medications, and mode of delivery. Endpoints in fetal outcomes included the incidence of preterm labor, stillbirth, and birth weight. There was no difference in nonvalvular baseline characteristics of the two groups, with the exception of a higher frequency of abortions in the VHD group.

Analysis of maternal outcomes revealed that, in aggregate, there was an advance of at least one functional class in 62% of patients with VHD, occurring most frequently in the second trimester (**202, 203**). None of the controls developed CHF.

The patients with VHD were also statistically more likely to develop arrhythmias, require cardiac medications, and hospitalization. There was no statistical difference in mortality. The single death in the two groups occurred in a woman with severe aortic stenosis and aortic coarctation 10 days following successful abdominal delivery while undergoing aortic valve replacement surgery. The relevance of her pregnancy to her death is uncertain. Regarding neonatal outcomes, a statistically significant increase in preterm delivery, intrauterine growth retardation, and a lower birth weight was seen in women with VHD compared to controls.

**203** Change in New York Heart Association (NYHA) functional class between first visit and follow-up during pregnancy in patients with predominant aortic and pulmonic valve disease. Circles: mild aortic stenosis; squares: moderate aortic stenosis; diamonds: severe aortic stenosis; triangles: pulmonic stenosis. Open symbols: NYHA functional class I on presentation; closed symbols: NYHA functional class II on presentation; dotted diamonds: NYHA functional class III on presentation. (Adapted from Hameed A, Karaalp IS, Tummala PP, *et al.* (2001). The effect of valvular heart disease on maternal and fetal outcome of pregnancy. *Journal of the American College of Cardiology* **37**:893–899.)

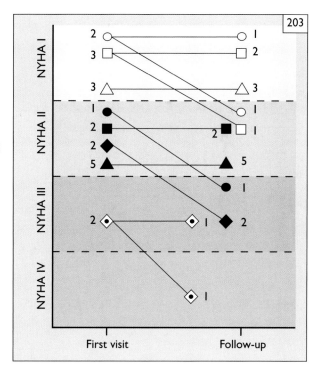

Subgroup analysis of specific valve lesions is limited by the relatively small sample size, but it appears that the outcomes of patients with mild mitral stenosis (MS), mild aortic stenosis (AS), and any degree of pulmonic stenosis (PS) did not differ from those of controls. Patients with more severe degrees of MS and AS, however, were clearly disadvantaged. *Tables 32* and *33* list lesions felt to be high and low risk, respectively, by the American Heart Association (AHA).

## Management guidelines for specific lesions

These recommendations were adapted from the most recently published guidelines from the AHA/American College of Cardiology (ACC) (Bonow *et al.*, 1998).

### MITRAL STENOSIS

As noted in the study by Hameed *et al.* (2001), most patients with mitral stenosis (MS) can be managed conservatively. Since rheumatic heart disease is still the most common etiology for MS in this age group, secondary prevention of rheumatic fever with penicillin should be continued throughout pregnancy. Pulmonary and systemic venous congestion should be managed with the lowest possible doses of diuretics to avoid hypoperfusion of the placenta. Beta-blockers should be used to control tachycardia and allow for increased left ventricular (LV) filling. Some authorities recommend β1 selective agents (e.g. metoprolol, atenolol) to avoid possible inhibition of myometrial contractility. If moderate or severe MS is diagnosed prior to pregnancy, consideration of percutaneous mitral balloon valvuloplasty should be considered. If a patient develops class III or IV CHF during pregnancy despite intensive medical management, valvuloplasty at a center with considerable experience should be considered. Fetal radiation exposure can be minimized by using echocardiography or minimal fluoroscopy (<2 minutes) with pelvic and abdominal shielding to guide the procedure. Surgical closed commissurotomy, employed for many years in developing countries, is another option.

### MITRAL REGURGITATION

Mitral valve prolapse (MVP) is the most common etiology of pathologic mitral regurgitation (MR) in pregnancy. The classic auscultatory signs may be masked by the decreased SVR and elevated blood volume of pregnancy. As mentioned in reference to mitral stenosis above, diuretic use should be minimized. Vasodilators should be employed only in the context of coexisting hypertension. Angiotensin-converting enzyme (ACE) inhibitors are contraindicated because of their teratogenic potential. Hydralazine is the preferred vasodilating agent. Surgery is indicated in cases of acute severe MR related to mechanical causes such as a ruptured chordae or papillary muscle. In light of the long life expectancy

---

**Table 32** Valvular heart lesions associated with high maternal and/or fetal risk during pregnancy

Severe AS with or without symptoms

AR with NYHA functional Class III–IV symptoms

MS with NYHA functional Class II–IV symptoms

MR with NYHA functional Class III–IV symptoms

Aortic and/or mitral valve disease resulting in severe pulmonary hypertension (pulmonary pressure >75% of systemic pressure)

Aortic and/or mitral valve disease with severe LV dysfunction (EF <0.40)

Mechanical prosthetic valve requiring anticoagulation

AR in Marfan syndrome

AR: aortic regurgitation; AS: aortic stenosis; EF: ejection fraction; LV: left ventricular; MR: mitral regurgitation; MS: mitral stenosis; NYHA: New York Heart Association. (Adapted from Bonow RO, Carabello B, de Leon AC Jr, *et al.* (1998). ACC/AHA guidelines for the management of patients with valvular heart disease. *Journal of the American College of Cardiology* **32**:1486–1588.)

of child-bearing women and the problems of anticoagulation in pregnancy, valve repair is strongly preferred over replacement.

## AORTIC STENOSIS

Congenital malformation of the valve (e.g. bicuspid valve) is the most common etiology of aortic stenosis (AS). If moderate or severe AS is recognized prior to conception, prophylactic valvuloplasty or valve repair should be seriously considered. As in MS, patients with normally functioning ventricles can nearly always be managed with intensive surveillance and judicious use of medications. Angina, syncope, or heart failure should prompt consideration of percutaneous aortic balloon valvotomy or surgery during pregnancy. It too should be performed in a center experienced in the technique. Because of the association between bicuspid aortic valves and cystic medial necrosis, the physician should remain vigilant for symptoms and signs of aortic dissection.

## AORTIC REGURGITATION

Analogous to MR, most patients with aortic regurgitation (AR) can be managed with judicious doses of diuretics and, if hypertension is present, vasodilator therapy with hydralazine. Consideration of surgery should be prompted only by class III or IV CHF despite intensive therapy by experienced physicians. Surgical criteria based on end-systolic and end-diastolic dimensions do not apply to pregnant women because of their obligate increase in total blood volume.

## PULMONIC STENOSIS

Isolated PS, a relatively rare entity, rarely causes problems as evidenced by the data of Hameed *et al.* (2001), and hence does not usually merit any intervention. However, when seen as a component of a larger syndrome of cyanotic heart disease, it may profoundly affect maternal and fetal outcomes. Patients with cyanotic heart disease should ideally be informed of the risks of pregnancy prior to conception and should be managed by experts in congenital heart disease.

## TRICUSPID VALVE DISEASE

Common etiologies in women of child-bearing age include Epstein's anomaly, tricuspid atresia, endocarditis, myxomatous proliferation, and carcinoid. Similar to PS, tricuspid disease alone rarely requires intervention during pregnancy. However, as part of a more complex congenital heart disease, it may require a very sophisticated approach best handled by a dedicated team.

## Endocarditis prophylaxis

According to the AHA guidelines, uncomplicated vaginal delivery in the absence of known infection is not a condition requiring antibiotic prophylaxis. As an exception, antibiotics are cited as optional in high-risk patients including those with prosthetic heart valves, prior endocarditis, complex congenital heart disease, or a surgically constructed systemic-pulmonary conduit. However, there is no consensus regarding this issue and many physicians routinely administer prophylactic antibiotics.

---

**Table 33** Valvular heart lesions associated with low maternal and fetal risk during pregnancy

Asymptomatic AS with low mean gradient(<50 mmHg [6.7 kPa]) in presence of normal LV systolic function (EF >0.50)

NYHA functional Class I or II AR with normal LV systolic function

NYHA functional Class I or II MR with normal LV systolic function

MVP with no MR or with mild to moderate MR and with normal LV systolic function

Mild to moderate MS (MVA >1.5cm$^2$, gradient <5 mmHg [0.7 kPa]) without severe pulmonary hypertension

Mild to moderate pulmonary valve stenosis

AR: aortic regurgitation; AS: aortic stenosis; EF: ejection fraction; LV: left ventricular; MR: mitral regurgitation; MS: mitral stenosis; MVA: mitral valve area; MVP: mitral valve prolapse; NYHA: New York Heart Association. (Adapted from Bonow RO, Carabello B, de Leon AC Jr, *et al.* (1998). ACC/AHA guidelines for the management of patients with valvular heart disease. *Journal of the American College of Cardiology* **32**:1486–1588.)

## Cardiac valve surgery

Open heart surgery with cardiopulmonary bypass must be considered a last resort given the challenge of providing adequate uteroplacental perfusion and the consequent risk to the fetus. It is obviously greatly preferable to pursue surgery either prior to conception or following delivery. As noted above, the principal indication is refractory pulmonary congestion or severe low output state despite maximal medical therapy and after consideration of percutaneous techniques. Because of the expected longevity of the patients, the hemodynamic strain on prostheses (**204, 205**), and the difficulties of anticoagulation (see below), a special premium is placed on efforts to repair valves.

## Anticoagulation

Patients with mechanical heart valve prostheses require anticoagulation. Unfortunately, there are little prospective data to guide recommendations regarding the appropriate level of anticoagulation and the ideal anticoagulation regimen does not exist (Iturbe-Alessio *et al.*, 1986; Sbarouni and Oakley, 1994). As noted below in more detail, heparin is safer for the fetus, but is inferior to warfarin in preventing valve-related thromboembolic events. The recommendations of the AHA are displayed in *Tables 34* and *35*.

### WARFARIN

This anticoagulant is classified as pregnancy category 'X' in light of its ability to cross the placenta and its association with spontaneous abortion, prematurity, stillbirth, cerebral hemorrhage, and embryopathy. The incidence of teratogenicity appears to be between 4% and 10%, with a maximal exposure risk occurring between gestational weeks 6 and 10. The risk of pregnancy-related complications appears to be dose dependent, with significantly increased risk at daily doses >5 mg (Cotrufo *et al.*, 2002). Low-dose aspirin is recommended as adjuvant therapy by the AHA.

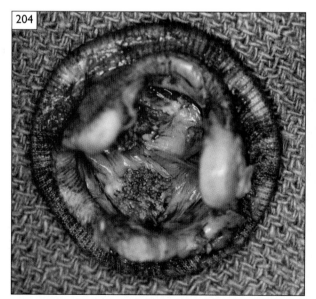
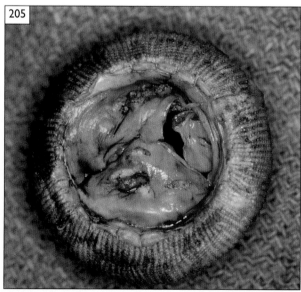

**204, 205** Degenerated bioprosthetic valve excised from a female patient who desired to avoid anticoagulants during her childbearing years. She underwent repeat valve replacement with a mechanical valve subsequent to the birth of her last child. **204** Inflow view. **205** Outflow view (note valve struts). (Courtesy of John Sanders, MD.)

HEPARIN

In recognition of its exclusion from the placental circulation, heparin has been considered safe in pregnant women. However, it is not free of risk. It is associated with sterile abscesses, osteoporosis, thrombocytopenia, and bleeding. Furthermore, based on case reports and registries of women with older generation (more thrombotic) valves without weight-based dosing, there has been a 12–24% risk of thromboembolic complications. Low-molecular weight heparin offers a number of potential advantages including less protein binding (hence more predictable anticoagulation), less thrombocytopenia, and greater ease of administration while still not crossing the placenta. However, there are no data regarding efficacy in pregnant women with prosthetic valves. Neither warfarin nor heparin is contraindicated in breast-feeding women.

**Table 34** Recommendations for anticoagulation during pregnancy in patients with mechanical prosthetic valves: weeks 1–35

| Indication | Class |
|---|---|
| The decision whether to use heparin during the first trimester or to continue oral anticoagulation throughout pregnancy should be made after full discussion with the patient and her partner; if she chooses to change to heparin for the first trimester, she should be made aware that heparin is less safe for her, with a higher risk of both thrombosis and bleeding, and that any risk to the mother also jeopardizes the baby* | I |
| High-risk women (a history of thromboembolism or an older generation mechanical prosthesis in the mitral position) who choose not to take warfarin during the first trimester should receive continuous unfractionated heparin IV in dose to prolong the midinterval (6 hours after dosing) aPTT to 2–3 times control. Transition to warfarin can occur thereafter | I |
| In patients receiving warfarin, INR should be maintained between 2.0 and 3.0 with the lowest possible dose of warfarin, and low-dose aspirin should be added | IIa |
| Women at low risk (no history of thromboembolism, newer low-profile prosthesis) may be managed with adjusted dose subcutaneous heparin( 17,500–20,000 U BID) to prolong the midinterval (6 hours after dosing) aPTT to 2–3 times control | IIb |

* From the European Society of Cardiology Guidelines for Prevention of Thromboembolic Events in Valvular Heart Disease. aPTT: actived partial thromboplastin time; INR: international normalized ratio. (Adapted from Bonow RO, Carabello B, de Leon AC Jr, et al. (1998). ACC/AHA guidelines for the management of patients with valvular heart disease. *Journal of the American College of Cardiology* **32**:1486–1588.)

**Table 35** Recommendations for anticoagulation during pregnancy in patients with mechanical prosthetic valves: after the 36th week

| Indication | Class |
|---|---|
| Warfarin should be stopped no later than week 36 and heparin substituted in anticipation of labor | IIa |
| If labor begins during treatment with warfarin a cesarian section should be performed | IIa |
| In the absence of significant bleeding, heparin can be resumed 4–6 hours after delivery and warfarin begun orally | IIa |

(Adapted from Bonow RO, Carabello B, de Leon AC Jr, et al. (1998). ACC/AHA guidelines for the management of patients with valvular heart disease. *Journal of the American College of Cardiology* **32**:1486–1588.)

## References

Bonow RO, Carabello B, de Leon AC Jr, *et al.* (1998). ACC/AHA guidelines for the management of patients with valvular heart disease: a report of the American College of Cardiology/American Heart Association Task Force on Practice Guidelines (Committee on Management of Patients with Valvular Heart Disease). *Journal of the American College of Cardiology* **32**:1486–1588.

Cotrufo M, De Feo M, De Santo LS, *et al.* (2002). Risk of warfarin during pregnancy with mechanical valve prostheses. *Obstetrics and Gynecology* **99**(1):35–40.

Hameed A, Karaalp IS, Tummala PP, *et al.* (2001). The effect of valvular heart disease on maternal and fetal outcome of pregnancy. *Journal of the American College of Cardiology* **37**:893–899.

Iturbe-Alessio I, Fonseca MC, Mutchinik O, *et al.* (1986). Risks of anticoagulant therapy in pregnant women with artificial heart valves. *New England Journal of Medicine* **315**:1390–1393.

Sbarouni E, Oakley CM (1994). Outcome of pregnancy in women with valve prostheses. *British Heart Journal* **71**:196–201.

# Chapter Twenty-One

# Valvular Heart Disease in the Elderly

## General considerations

### EPIDEMIOLOGY

The aging of the Western population is a frequently published observation. By virtue of an increase in life expectancy and a declining birth rate in developed countries, the elderly comprise an increasing proportion of society. In the US, the population exceeding the age of 80 was 6.9 million in 1990. By the year 2050, this age group is expected to number 25 million. It is instructive to note that the average life expectancy at age 80 years is 6.9 years for men and 8.7 years for women. This demographic shift and the declining incidence of rheumatic fever mean that an increasing proportion of patients with valvular heart disease (VHD) will be elderly. It is important that physicians appreciate the special considerations in diagnosing and managing VHD in the elderly.

### EFFECT OF NORMAL AGING

There is considerable individual variation in biologic age among individuals of the same chronological age. However, in general, in advanced old age, patients lose the functional reserve of many organ systems (Pretre *et al.*, 2000). This reserve, representing the difference between daily function in health and the minimum level of function required to maintain homeostasis, becomes progressively smaller. Practically, this means that the elderly are much more vulnerable to the physiologic burdens created by VHD and to the stresses of surgical intervention.

### PREVALENCE OF COMORBIDITIES

In addition to the problems of normal aging, many elderly patients with VHD are burdened with independent chronic illnesses. In patients over 80 years old these include coronary artery disease (15–25%), renal insufficiency (5–10%), peripheral vascular disease (2–10%), cerebrovascular disease (5–25%), hypertension (20–30%), and diabetes (10–20%) (Pretre *et al.*, 2000). A comorbidity of particular concern to the cardiovascular surgeon is the presence of atherosclerosis and calcification of the aortic arch. Prevalence data based on intraoperative and/or epiaortic echocardiography have documented that 20% of patients >75 years old have protruding atheroma in this location (Katz *et al.*, 1992).

## Impact of aging on the presentation and evaluation

### AORTIC VALVE DISEASE

*Aortic sclerosis*

Defined as thickening without hemodynamic stenosis, aortic sclerosis is a common finding in the elderly. Population-based samples suggest a prevalence of 26% over the age of 65 and 48% in individuals older than 85 years. It is recognized incidentally on physical exam as a soft, systolic murmur or by 2D echocardiography. No symptoms should be attributed to this finding because it is functionally benign. However, it is clinically important as a marker for atherosclerosis and may progress to aortic stenosis (AS) (Stewart *et al.*, 1997).

*Aortic stenosis*

Calcific aortic valve disease is the most common valvular lesion seen in the elderly. Less common etiologies in this age group include rheumatic heart disease and degeneration of congenitally bicuspid valves (Hinchman and Otto, 1999). Hemodynamically significant AS is present in 2–9% of those over age 65 years. In this age group, the clinician must be vigilant for atypical presentations of all diseases. Rather than the classic presenting symptoms of angina, syncope, and heart failure, the elderly with AS often complain of failing exercise capacity, exertional dyspnea, or dizziness. Because of the increased prevalence of coronary artery disease, the elderly may present with angina at mild or moderate degrees of AS. In some cases, the hemodynamic load is not exposed until a patient develops an acute illness such as sepsis or profound anemia. Under-recognition of AS in the elderly is fostered by the tendency of patients to attribute their initially mild symptoms to normal aging and by the broad differential posed by fatigue and dizziness.

Pitfalls in the physical exam of elderly patients with AS include the prevalence of soft systolic murmurs despite severe stenosis, the prevalence of benign systolic murmurs, and the presence of rapid carotid upstrokes caused by noncompliant vessels.

A special consideration in the laboratory evaluation of AS not specifically addressed in Chapter 4 includes the nearly absolute need for angiography prior to valve surgery because of the frequent coexistence of obstructive coronary artery disease. Additionally, estimated aortic valve area must be interpreted in the context of the patient's size and physical activity (Hinchman and Otto, 1999). An aortic valve area of 0.75 cm$^2$ may be perfectly adequate for a sedentary, 45 kg (100 lb) , 80-year-old female but severely stenotic for a 90 kg (200 lb), 1.85 m (6 foot), active, 70-year-old male.

## Aortic regurgitation

Regurgitation of the aortic valve (AR) is quite common in patients >65 years. Population-based studies suggest a prevalence of AR of 20–30%, but it is usually mild and not functionally significant (Lindroos *et al.*, 1993). In this age group, the mechanism is most commonly aortic sclerosis or aortic root dilatation resulting from hypertension or atherosclerosis. While much of the discussion in Chapter 5 applies to the elderly, it is controversial whether surgery should be pursued in the very elderly in the absence of symptoms (i.e. in asymptomatic patients with left ventricular [LV] dilatation or diminished ejection fraction). Also open to debate is the practice of treating asymptomatic patients with severe AR and elevated systolic pressure with nifedipine. The clinical trial establishing its usefulness enrolled younger patients (Scognamiglio *et al.*, 1994), and the results may not be generalizable to elderly patients.

## MITRAL VALVE

### Mitral annular calcification

This degenerative process is seen with increasing frequency with advancing age. While it may be seen on fluoroscopy or chest radiographs, echocardio-graphy is more sensitive (**206, 207**). Its prevalence has been reported as approximately 20% in the seventh decade of life, 33% in the eighth decade, 62% in the ninth decade, and 100% among those rare individuals living more than 100 years (Aronow *et al.*, 1990). Its pathogenesis is obscure but it may parallel that of AS discussed in Chapter 4.

Mitral regurgitation (MR) is present in approximately 50% of patients with mitral annular calcification (MAC); it is moderate or severe in 20–33% (Labovitz *et al.*, 1985). In rare instances, mitral stenosis (MS) develops. Atrial enlargement and conduction defects are frequently associated findings. Electrical complications of mitral annular calcification include atrial fibrillation, complete heart block, and sudden cardiac death. Vascular complications include an increased incidence of thromboembolic stroke and myocardial infarction (Aranow *et al.*, 1990; 1998).

### Mitral stenosis

Obstruction of the mitral valve is a rare condition in the elderly since most MS is rheumatic in origin and usually presents earlier in life. However, as mentioned above, MAC may progress centripetally to affect the leaflets. As in younger patients, the elderly with MS usually present with congestive heart failure (CHF). However, in contrast, the typical signs (loud $S_1$, opening snap, diastolic rumble) are present in <50% (Hammer *et al.*, 1978).

### Mitral regurgitation

MR is a common finding in the elderly but is usually mild and rarely requires intervention. As described in Chapter 9, valve leakage may result from distortion of anatomic structures ranging from the leaflet tips to the LV wall. In this age group, the most common etiologies are myxomatous disease (sometimes accompanied by ruptured chordae), MAC with its attendant loss of annular systolic contraction, and ischemic cardiomyopathy with dilatation of the ventricle and annulus preventing coaptation of normal leaflets (Hinchman and Otto, 1999). Symptoms and physical exam findings are influenced more by the specific mechanism than the age of the patient.

## TRICUSPID AND PULMONIC VALVE DISEASE

Mild tricuspid regurgitation (TR) and pulmonic regurgitation (PR) are progressively more common with advancing age but are rarely hemodynamically significant. While myxomatous degeneration, endo-carditis, and a myriad other conditions may lead to regurgitant right-sided valves, pulmonary hypertension is the most common cause. Once elevated pulmonary pressures are recognized, the clinician should search for a treatable cause (e.g. ischemic heart disease, left-sided valvular disease, chronic hypoxemia, veno-occlusive disease, chronic obstructive pulmonary disease [COPD], diffuse parenchymal lung disease, chronic occult thrombo-embolic disease).

INFECTIVE ENDOCARDITIS

Coincident with the aging of the population and the increasing prevalence of prosthetic valves in the elderly, there has been a shift in the average age of patients with infective endocarditis (IE) (Warner *et al.*, 1996). A special challenge in the elderly is the tendency for patients, their families, and sometimes their physicians, to attribute nonspecific symptoms such as weight loss and fatigue to aging. For this reason, the diagnosis is often delayed. Another special consideration is the more limited sensitivity of transthoracic echocardiography in this age group due to obesity, COPD, valve calcification, and prosthetic valves. Transesophageal echocardiography (TEE) should be entertained as the initial procedure. The bacteriology also differs in the elderly, since the bowel and bladder are more frequently the source of infection. The most common organisms are *Staphylococcus aureus*, group D streptococci, and enterococci. Another interesting difference in the elderly is the less frequent occurrence of embolic events, perhaps due to the nature of the common pathogens (Selton-Suty *et al.*, 1997).

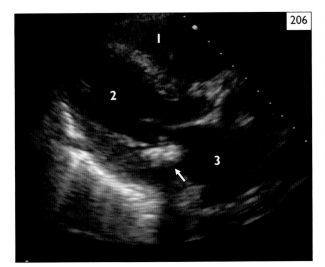
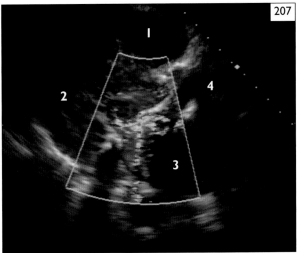

**206, 207** Posterior mitral annular calcification associated with mitral regurgitation. **206** 2D parasternal long axis view. Note the thickened and densely echogenic character of the posterior annulus (arrow) with acoustic shadowing (black area) behind the annulus. **207** Doppler color imaging demonstrating a wide jet of regurgitant flow into the left atrium. 1: right ventricle; 2: left ventricle; 3: left atrium; 4: aortic root.

## Special considerations in valve surgery in the elderly
### WEIGHING RISKS AND BENEFITS

Although it is difficult to isolate the contribution of age alone from the frequently accompanying comorbidities, most risk scores consider age >80 years as a significant risk factor. This is true of the French score (208) (Roques *et al.*, 1995). This increased risk of mortality and morbidity must be balanced against the expected benefit. Since a mortality benefit is difficult to demonstrate in this age group, it is symptom and functional improvement that must be considered. Operations for asymptomatic conditions or in patients whose quality of life is determined by noncardiovascular conditions such as dementia, advanced cancer or end-stage renal disease should not be pursued. In addition, patient effort and cooperation with the rehabilitation plan are essential to a positive surgical outcome. In some cases, a compromise approach of less complete surgery with lower risk may be appropriate. In all cases, the patient and their family should be fully informed of the operative risks and realistic benefit. Applying their own values and risk tolerance, they can actively participate in decision making. The patient should be encouraged to discuss end-of-life care and to appoint a surrogate decision maker.

### PREOPERATIVE INVESTIGATIONS

As discussed above, the prevalence of advanced coronary atherosclerosis justifies routine coronary angiography before all valve surgery in this age group. For the same reason, 2D and Doppler ultrasound of the carotid arteries should be considered prior to surgery. Symptomatic or bilateral high-grade stenosis is probably best treated before or during cardiac surgery. Knowledge of asymptomatic high-grade disease may impact the choice of bypass perfusion pressure or the decision to employ systemic hypothermia (Pretre *et al.*, 2000).

### CHOICE OF PROSTHESIS

In the aortic position, most surgeons use bioprosthetic valves in order to avoid the hazards of anticoagulation in this age group. The downside of bioprostheses in younger patients, their limited durability, is generally irrelevant in patients >80 years old. However, another distinguishing feature of bioprosthetic valves, their slightly increased transvalvular gradient, may be relevant in a patient with an annulus <21 mm, usually a small female. In these individuals, a properly sized bioprosthetic valve may result in significant postoperative obstruction (known as patient–valve mismatch). Possible solutions include a bileaflet mechanical prosthesis with good flow characteristics and very carefully monitoring of prothrombin times, a lower resistance stentless bioprosthetic valve which has lesser gradients, or surgically enlarging the annulus. Each of these approaches poses competing benefits and risks.

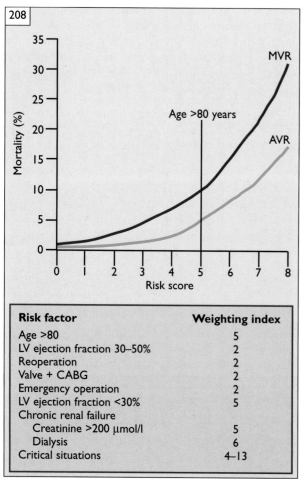

| Risk factor | Weighting index |
|---|---|
| Age >80 | 5 |
| LV ejection fraction 30–50% | 2 |
| Reoperation | 2 |
| Valve + CABG | 2 |
| Emergency operation | 2 |
| LV ejection fraction <30% | 5 |
| Chronic renal failure | |
|     Creatinine >200 µmol/l | 5 |
|     Dialysis | 6 |
| Critical situations | 4–13 |

**208** Mortality rates of aortic and mitral valve surgery according to the cumulated risk score. Critical situations include urgent operations (acute aortic dissection, postinfarction ventricular septal defect, or papillary muscle avulsion) and necessity to operate within 48 hours after myocardial infarction. AVR: aortic valve replacement; CABG: coronary artery bypass graft; LV: left ventricular; MVR: mitral valve replacement. (Adapted from Roques F, Gabrielle F, Michel P, *et al.* (1995). Quality of care in adult heart surgery: proposal for a self-assessment approach based on a French multicenter study. *European Journal of Cardiothoracic Surgery* **9**:433–439.)

In the mitral position, most surgeons again select bioprostheses to avoid anticoagulation. However, they are technically more difficult to implant in patients with a normal sized ventricle, and the stents may extend into the left ventricular outflow tract and cause subaortic stenosis. For this reason, a low profile mechanical prosthesis is sometimes selected.

RESULTS

In modern series, the reported mortality rates for isolated aortic valve replacement (AVR) in octogenarians has ranged from 5 to 10% compared to 2 to 3% for younger patients (Gehlot *et al.*, 1996; Akins *et al.*, 1997). When coronary artery bypass graft (CABG) is required in addition, inhospital mortality climbs to 15–20%. However, those who survive do well, often with a dramatic improvement in function and quality of life (Olsson *et al.*, 1996). Survival curves from a large nonrandomized series are displayed in **209**. Postoperative survival is similar to an age-matched, unselected population.

The results of mitral valve surgery depend largely upon whether or not the valve is repairable. Myxomatous valves with prolapsing or flail leaflets are well suited to repair, with the possible addition of an annular ring to reduce the increased antero-posterior diameter of the annulus. Heavy MAC makes sewing very difficult. In patients >65 years old undergoing mitral valve repair, an operative mortality rate of 4% and a 1-year survival of 90% have been reported (Bolling *et al.*, 1996). However, the results of mitral valve replacement are not as encouraging. A nation-wide UK registry reported a 10% 30-day mortality rate and 1-, 3-, and 5-year survival rates of 80%, 64%, and 41%, respectively (Asimakopouios *et al.*, 1997). As discussed in Chapter 9, preservation of subvalvular apparatus is associated with better outcomes and should be attempted. There are no data concerning quality of life in this age stratum.

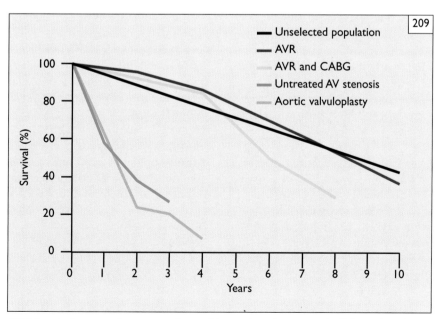

**209** Survival rates of octogenarians with aortic valve stenosis. AV: aortic valve; AVR: aortic valve replacement; CABG: coronary artery bypass graft. (Adapted from Gehlot A, Mullany CJ, Ilstrup D, *et al.*, (1996). Aortic valve replacement in patients aged 80 years and older: early and long-term results. *Journal of Thoracic and Cardiovascular Surgery* **111**:1026–1036.)

## References

Akins CW, Daggett WM, Vlahakes GJ, *et al.* (1997). Cardiac operations in patients 80 years old and older. *Annals of Thoracic Surgery* 64:606–614.

Aronow WS, Koenigsberg M, Kronzon I, *et al.* (1990). Association of mitral annular calcium with new thrombotic stroke and cardiac events at 39-month follow-up in elderly patients. *American Journal of Cardiology* 65:1511–1512.

Aronow WS, Ahn C, Kronzon I, Gutstein H (1998). Association of mitral annular calcium with new thromboembolic stroke at 44-month follow-up of 2148 persons, mean age 81 years. *American Journal of Cardiology* 81:105–106.

Asimakopouios G, Edwards MB, Brannan J, *et al.* (1997). Survival and cause of death after mitral valve replacement in patients 80 years and over: collective results from the UK heart valve registry. *European Journal of Cardiothoracic Surgery* 11:922–928.

Bolling SF, Deeb GM, Bach DS (1996). Mitral valve reconstruction in elderly ischemic patients. *Chest* 109:35–40.

Gehlot A, Mullany CJ, Ilstrup D, *et al.* (1996). Aortic valve replacement in patients aged 80 years and older: early and long-term results. *Journal of Thoracic and Cardiovascular Surgery* 111:1026–1036.

Hammer WJ, Roberts WC, deLeon AC (1978). 'Mitral stenosis' secondary to combined 'massive' mitral annular calcific deposits and small, hypertrophied left ventricles. Hemodynamic documentation in four patients. *American Journal of Medicine* 64: 371–376.

Hinchman DA, Otto CM (1997). Cardiovascular disease in the elderly. *Cardiology Clinics* 17(1):137–158.

Hinchman DA, Otto CM (1999). Valvular disease in the elderly. *Cardiology Clinics* 17(1):137–158.

Katz ES, Tunick PA, Rusinek H, *et al.* (1992). Protruding aortic atheroma predict stroke in elderly patients undergoing cardiopulmonary bypass: experience with intraoperative transesophageal echocardiography. *Journal of the American College of Cardiology* 20:70–77.

Labovitz AJ, Nelson JG, Windhorst DM, *et al.* (1985). Frequency of mitral valve dysfunction from mitral annular calcium as detected by Doppler echocardiography. *American Journal of Cardiology* 55:133–137.

Lindroos M, Kupari M, Heikkila J, *et al.* (1993). Prevalence of aortic valve abnormalities in the elderly: an echocardiographic study of a random population sample. *Journal of the American College of Cardiology* 21:1220–1225.

Olsson M, Janfjall H, Orth-Gomer K, *et al.* (1996). Quality of life in octogenarians after valve replacement due to aortic stenosis. A prospective comparison with younger patients. *European Heart Journal* 17:583–589.

Pretre R, Turino MI (2000). Cardiac valve surgery in the octogenarian. *Heart* 83(1):116–121.

Roques F, Gabrielle F, Michel P, *et al.* (1995). Quality of care in adult heart surgery: proposal for a self-assessment approach based on a French multicenter study. *European Journal of Cardiothoracic Surgery* 9:433–439.

Scognamiglio R, Rahimtoola SH, Fasoli G, *et al.* (1994). Nifedipine in asymptomatic patients with severe aortic regurgitation and normal left ventricular function. *New England Journal of Medicine* 331:689–694.

Selton-Suty C, Hoen B, Grentzinger A, *et al.* (1997). Clinical and bacteriological characteristics of infective endocarditis in the elderly. *Heart* 77:260–263.

Stewart BF, Siscovick D, Lind BK, *et al.* (1997). Clinical factors associated with calcific aortic valve disease. Cardiovascular Health Study. *Journal of the American College of Cardiology* 29:630–634.

Warner GS, Schulz R, Fuchs JB, *et al.* (1996). Infective endocarditis in the elderly in the era of transesophageal echocardiography: clinical features compared to younger patients. *American Journal of Medicine* 100:90–97.

# Chapter Twenty-Two

# Quality Improvement in Valvular Heart Disease

## Introduction

Improving the quality of health care is the responsibility of all parties involved. This includes the individual clinician who strives to work carefully and thoughtfully, to generate hypotheses to explain unexpected events, and to use innovation and creativity when appropriate. It also involves basic scientists studying molecular and cellular processes in the pathogenesis of valvular heart disease (VHD) and the pharmaceutical and medical device manufacturing industry working to develop better products. Improvement also relies on the efforts of clinical work teams (e.g. coronary care staff, operating room staff, cardiac catheterization laboratory staff) to streamline processes and coordinate individual efforts. At the institutional and national level, improving quality in VHD relies on systematic data collection and administrative support of quality improvement.

## Outcome measures

Traditional outcome measures, cited frequently in this text, consist of procedure-related death and postoperative survival rates. However, meaningful measures of clinical results include additional issues of importance to the patient, such as ability to perform daily activities, satisfaction with health care, social functioning, and emotional well-being (Birkmeyer et al., 2001). One way of combining these measures is through the use of a clinical value compass in which outcomes are plotted along the following four axes: functional health, patient satisfaction, cost, and clinical outcome (Nelson et al., 1996). Many other standardized instruments are available for this purpose.

## Examining variation

One approach to identifying opportunities for improvement is to study variation. In VHD, this has been done at both national and international levels. The Dartmouth Atlas of Cardiovascular Health Care has documented variation in the nationwide rate of aortic valve replacement over time. On a per Medicare enrollee basis, the rate of this procedure doubled from 1988 to 1997 (Wennberg et al., 1999). Much of this increase occurred in the very elderly. There was also a fourfold geographical variation in aortic valve replacement (AVR) rates, ranging from 0.4/1000 to 1.6/1000 Medicare enrollees. Another example of outcome analysis is the data published by the Northern New England Cardiovascular Disease Study Group (NNE). This regional, voluntary collaboration of tertiary hospitals has prospectively collected data regarding cardiovascular care since 1987. In Canada, outcome researchers recently compared risk adjusted in-hospital mortality for mitral and aortic valve surgery and found considerable interprovincial variation (Hassan et al., 2004).

While this variation may represent an opportunity for improvement, it does not provide very specific direction. It may represent true differences in populations, uncertainty in 'best practice', or failure of the medical community to disseminate knowledge successfully.

## Approaches to improving results

There are many potential avenues to improving VHD care. This section will address only a few. At the level of basic science, laboratory investigations can improve understanding of the subcellular mechanisms involved in aortic stenosis, myxomatous valve disease, and bioprosthetic valve failure. Both *ex-vivo* and *in-vivo* animal studies can be used to test new medications and devices. Successful animal studies can be followed by phase I and phase II clinical studies. Finally, randomized clinical trials in patients can be performed with permission from regulatory bodies. These methods are the traditional forms of medical research.

Other approaches include applying the results of different epidemiologic and clinical trial data in a formal clinical decision analysis. An example of this is a Markov model to simulate the occurrence of valve-related events and life expectancy in patients undergoing AVR (Birkmeyer *et al.*, 2000a). This approach allows reasoned predictions and the ability to vary assumptions (sensitivity analysis) regarding clinical scenarios unlikely to be tested in randomized clinical trials.

Another avenue of quality improvement is to examine registry data and attempt to correct for known differences in risk. This allows analysis of large, prospectively collected databases (Birkmeyer *et al.*, 2000b; Roques *et al.*, 1995). However, like all nonexperimental approaches, it has its critics. One topic of frequent debate is the specific patient factors which should be considered in risk adjustment.

To address the problem of incomplete dissemination of knowledge, an approach frequently employed is to publish practice guidelines, drafted by experts, based on clinical evidence, and endorsed by a respected peer group such as the subspecialty college or society. An example of this is the ACC/AHA guidelines found throughout this text. For a variety of reasons, a significant gap exists between clinical practice and published guidelines. The reasons include lack of awareness of their existence, disagreement with the recommendations, resentment over a perceived loss of autonomy, and skepticism regarding the intent of the guidelines (Cabana, 1999). As recently pointed out in the British surgical literature, there is an established methodology to developing clinical guidelines that unfortunately is not always followed. In addition, guidelines alone cannot be relied upon to address quality improvement in a community or institution (Andrews *et al.*, 2004).

Lastly, because a relationship between procedural volume and outcome has been observed in percutaneous cardiac intervention (Harjai *et al.*, 2004), coronary bypass surgery (Wennberg *et al.*, 1999; Peterson *et al.*, 2004), and the rate of mitral valve repair (Northrup *et al.*, 2003), the regionalization of challenging and high-risk surgery such as valve surgery into high volume centers has been suggested. However, there are insufficient data to support this proposal at present and it would create the problems of loss of continuity of care with regular physicians, distance from family when their support is needed, and possible economic strain on community hospitals.

## Conclusion

Quality improvement is the responsibility of all individuals involved in the care of patients with VHD. A variety of methods are available to define opportunities for improvement, including the study of variation and effort at many levels, from the subcellular to the institutional, to optimize patient outcomes.

## References

Andrews EJ, Redmond HP (2004). A review of clinical guidelines. *British Journal of Surgery* 91(8):956–964.

Birkmeyer N, Birkmeyer J, Tosteson A, *et al.* (2000a). Prosthetic valve type for patients undergoing AVR: a decision analysis. *Annals of Thoracic Surgery* 70:1946–1952.

Birkmeyer N, Marrin C, Morton J, *et al.* (2000b). Decreasing mortality for aortic and mitral valve replacement in Northern New England. *Annals of Thoracic Surgery* 70:732–737.

Birkmeyer NJ, O'Connor GT, Baldwin JC (2001). Aortic valve replacement: current clinical practice and opportunities for quality improvement. *Current Opinion in Cardiology* 16(2):152–157.

Cabana M, Rand C, Powe N, *et al.* (1999). Why don't physicians follow clinical practice guidelines? A framework for improvement. *Journal of the American Medical Association* 282:1458–1465.

Harjai KJ, Berman AD, Grines CL, *et al.* (2004). Impact of interventionalist volume, experience, and board certification on coronary angioplasty outcomes in the era of stenting. *American Journal of Cardiology* 94(4):421–426.

Hassan A, Quan H, Newman A, *et al.* for the Canadian Cardiovascular Outcomes Research Team (2004). Outcomes after aortic and mitral valve replacement surgery in Canada: 1994/95 to 1999/2000. *Canadian Journal of Cardiology* **20**(2):155–163.

Nelson E, Mohr J, Batalden P, *et al.* (1996). Improving health care, Part I: the clinical value compass. *Journal of Quality Improvement* **22**:243–258.

Northrup WF 3rd, Kshettry VR, DuBois KA (2003). Trends in mitral valve surgery in a large multisurgeon, multihospital practice, 1979–1999. *Journal of Heart Valve Disease* **12**(1):14–24.

Peterson ED, Coombs LP, DeLong ER, *et al.* (2004). Procedural volume as a marker of quality for CABG surgery. *Journal of the American Medical Association* **291**(2):195–201.

Nelson E, Mohr J, Batalden P, *et al.* (1996). Improving health care, Part I: the clinical value compass. *Journal of Quality Improvement* **22**:243–258.

Roques F, Gabrielle F, Michel P, *et al.* (1995). Quality of care in adult heart surgery: proposal for a self-assessment approach based on a French multicenter study. *European Journal of Cardiothoracic Surgery* **9**:433–439.

Wennberg D, Birkmeyer J, McAndrew CM (1999). The Dartmouth Atlas of Cardiovascular Health Care. Health Forum, AHA Press, Chicago, pp. 192–199.

# Chapter Twenty-Three

# Recent and Future Developments in Valvular Heart Disease

## Introduction

An increasingly sophisticated understanding of basic biologic science and continuing innovation in biomedical technology will continue to shape the evaluation and treatment of patients with valvular heart disease (VHD). In many instances, distinct technologies are competing to serve the same clinical purpose. Predicting which of these will prevail is difficult. The adaptation of new techniques and devices is determined by many factors, including efficacy, safety, cost, convenience, regulatory approval, ease of integration with existing technology, and timing of arrival on the market. Government regulators will play an important role. They must negotiate between the demand to provide access to new life-saving or life-improving technology and the obligation to protect the public from therapy that may have rare or very late-onset but grave complications. Finally, even the wealthiest societies will be unable to afford every advance in biomedical technology. Cost-effectiveness analysis will likely play an increasingly important role in government and private insurance coverage decisions. Obviously, those developments that both improve outcomes and save money will dominate. In this chapter, recent developments will be reviewed (Rahimtoola, 2005) and their implication for future clinical care will be considered.

## Biology and prevention

In the past several years, more sophisticated understanding has been achieved of the molecular mechanisms responsible for heart valve development and, in particular, the signaling pathways responsible for the transformation of endothelial cells to mesenchymal cells (Chang et al., 2004). Because some valve lesions (e.g. myxomatous mitral valve prolapse) resemble the embryonic proliferative phase of valve development, some investigators have suggested that dysregulation of embryonic angiogenic modulators may play a important mechanistic role in their development (Shworak, 2004).

Evidence supporting the hypothesis that aortic stenosis (AS) represents an inflammatory process paralleling that of atherosclerosis has continued to accumulate. As mentioned in Chapter 4, epidemiologic studies have documented the similar risk factors for the two conditions. At the cellular level, recent studies of stenotic valves have identified the presence of bone formation, inflammation, and neoangiogenesis. At the protein level, calcified AS has been associated with increased levels of C-reactive protein (Gerber et al., 2003a) and matrix metalloproteinases (Satta et al., 2003). In addition, there is evidence of active regulation of valve calcification by proteins known to participate in bone development (Rajamannan et al., 2003; Kaden et al.,

2004). At the level of transcription, increased heat shock protein-60 gene expression has been reported (Mazzone *et al.*, 2004). At the genomic level, the apolipoprotein E allele is overrepresented among patients with AS as compared to controls (Navaro *et al.*, 2003).

Another interesting basic development is the growing immunohistochemical parallels between the thoracic aortic tissue of patients with Marfan syndrome and those with bicuspid aortic valves. In both conditions, there are decreased extracellular levels of fibrillin, fibronectin, and tenascin. In addition, there is increased expression of matrix metalloproteinase-2 (Nataatmadja *et al.*, 2003). Similarly, immunohistochemical stains for fibrillin show a more diffuse and nonlaminar pattern in patients with mitral valve prolapse (MVP) compared to controls (Nasuti *et al.*, 2004).

As discussed in Chapter 9, idiopathic or ischemic-related left ventricular (LV) dilatation is a common cause of chronic mitral regurgitation (MR), in which the regurgitation is believed to represent mechanical dysfunction of a biologically normal valve. This concept has been challenged by the recent findings of increased deoxyribonucleic acid (DNA), glycoamino-glycans, and collagen in the explanted mitral valves of patients receiving transplants for dilated and ischemic cardiomyopathy (Grande-Allen *et al.*, 2005). The authors suggest that adverse loading conditions promote remodeling of the valve matrix.

The implications of these findings are that anti-inflammatory therapy may play an increasingly important role in the care of patients with mild and moderate AS. It is possible that localized gene therapy may eventually play a role in manipulation of the extracellular matrix of the ascending aorta and the mitral valve.

## Diagnosis and imaging techniques

In the arena of serum markers, the utility of natriuretic peptide levels was, not surprisingly, found to correlate with the severity of AS (Bergler-Klein *et al.*, 2004) and aortic regurgitation (AR) (Gerber *et al.*, 2003b). Furthermore, among patients who were asymptomatic, the levels of natriuretic peptides appears to help predict which patients will become symptomatic. Another serum marker, procalcitonin, was found to be elevated in those patients with suspected infective endocarditis in whom the diagnosis was later confirmed (Mueller *et al.*, 2004).

In a comparison of echocardiographic- and intracardiac catheter-derived measures of mitral valve area in mitral stenosis (MS), real-time three dimensional (RT3D) echocardiography demonstrated better reproducibility and agreement than pressure half-time, proximal isovelocity surface area (PISA), and planimetered two dimensional (2D) techniques (Zamorano *et al.*, 2004).

Another emerging technique, electron beam computed tomography (EBCT) has been proposed as a means of diagnosing AS. However, recent studiess have shown only 24% sensitivity of EBCT in comparison to echocardiography for detection of aortic valve disease (Walsh *et al.*, 2004). In contrast, the distinct multislice computed tomographic (MSCT) technique of three-dimensional volume quantification of aortic valve calcification was shown to correlate well with echocardiographic assessments of stenosis (Morgan-Hughes *et al.*, 2003). Multidetector computed tomography (MDCT) has also been successful in the detection of pannus formation on prosthetic heart valves (Teshima *et al.*, 2004). Another imaging technique with possible utility in prosthetic valve disease is transcranial Doppler, which has measured an increase in high intensity transit signals in patients with obstructed prosthetic heart valves.

In nuclear cardiology, positron emission tomography (PET) scanning was used to quantify the number of viable myocardial wall segments prior to mitral valve repair in chronic MR. Those patients with >5 (out of a total of 17) segments of viable myocardium had lower 6 month mortality than those with <5 segments (Pu *et al.*, 2003). Finally, cardiac magnetic resonance (CMR) has shown good correlation with echocardiography in the determination of transvalvular flow and aortic valve area (Caruthers *et al.*, 2003).

Based on these trends, one can expect continued exploration of serum markers for the diagnosis of, and as an aid in the timing of intervention in patients with heart valve disease. While echocardiography is hard to beat in terms of its relatively low cost, freedom from radiation, and portability, it is likely that CT and CMR will continue to develop niches of use. For the immediate future, they will likely be in circumstances where very accurate volume quantification is required and in patients with poor echocardiographic windows.

## Pharmacologic management

Until recently, there has been very little prospective human evidence upon which to base recommen-dations regarding endocarditis prophylaxis. However, a recent double blind, randomized clinical trial of antibiotic prophylaxis proved that amoxicillin reduced bacteremia following endotracheal intubation and dental work in children (Lockhart *et al.*, 2004). In another randomized trial, aspirin did not reduce the rate of embolization in patients with infective endocarditis (Chau *et al.*, 2003).

In the future, it is likely that statins (mentioned in Chapter 4) and angiotensin-converting enzyme (ACE) inhibitors will play a greater role in modifying the course of valvular heart disease. In addition, we can expect increasing refinement of the patient groups which benefit from antibiotic use to prevent endocarditis.

## Electrophysiologic techniques

In patients with functional MR due to LV dilatation and poor systolic function who also have QRS prolongation, cardiac resynchronization therapy (CRT) by biventricular pacing has been shown to improve function and mortality (MIRACLE and COMPANION trials). This is achieved in part by a reduction in MR. In addition, there is evidence that Doppler guided optimization of the atrioventricular (AV) delay in patients with pacemakers may improve net forward flow. In light of these findings, electrophysiologic techniques will continue to be used increasingly as an adjunct in the treatment of patients with functional MR and tricuspid regurgitation (TR).

## Percutaneous and surgical techniques

While randomized clinical trials (RCTs) are scarcer in surgical treatment than in pharmacologic therapy, two randomized surgical trials were recently reported. One single center trial compared the outcomes of patients randomized to a Starr–Edwards valve versus a St. Jude valve in follow-up reaching 8 years. There were no differences in survival or event-free survival (Murday *et al.*, 2003). The other recent surgical RCT compared the Carpentier–Edwards (CE) pericardial valve to the Toronto Stentless Prosthetic Valve (TSP). There was no difference in the primary end-point of LV mass regression, but the CE pericardial valve was associated with shorter bypass and cross-clamp times (Cohen *et al.*, 2002).

The Alfieri stitch is a surgical procedure used to reduce MR in patients in whom definitive repair is not possible, by suturing together the midpoints of the anterior and posterior leaflets of the mitral valve. Using an atrial trans-septal percutaneous technique, investigators used a new endovascular device to clip the anterior and posterior leaflets of adult pigs (St. Goar *et al.*, 2003). Another innovative endovascular approach to MR was recently reported. In a sheep model of dilated cardiomyopathy, a mitral annular constraint device was placed in the coronary sinus and thereby passed around the perimeter of the mitral valve. In an attempt to simulate the effect of surgical annulplasty, the annular circumference was reduced by an adjustable cable which pulled together anchors in the proximal and distal coronary sinus (Kaye *et al.*, 2003).

In the past, the magnitude of right ventricular outflow tract (RVOT) dilatation has limited the patients eligible for percutaneous valves. Recently, however, a larger stent has been developed and used successfully in a small number of patients with pulmonic regurgitation (Boudjemline *et al.*, 2004). On the left side of the heart, there have been six patients reported to date who have received percutaneously placed aortic valves. All have been end-stage, nonsurgical candidates. Five of six survived the operation. Three of the five died within 8 weeks but the short-term hemodynamic results were promising. In the five early survivors, aortic valve area increased from 0.49 cm$^2$ to 1.66 cm$^2$ and LV ejection fraction increased from 24% to 41% (Cribier *et al.*, 2004).

Though repair of leaky mitral valves is well established, repair of regurgitant aortic valves has been much more problematic. However, a series of 160 patients undergoing aortic valve repair was recently reported. The 7 year reoperation rate and survival rates were 15% and 89% respectively (Minakata *et al.*, 2004).

Finally, a radical approach to AS has been explored 'on the benchtop'. Intact human aortic valves were hemodynamically tested before and after surgical and chemical debridement. Mineral removal was measured by atomic absorption spectroscopy. Improvements in effective orifice area of up to 40% were seen (Ohashi *et al.*, 2004).

Thus, innovations are likely to continue, and it seems likely that patients will have an increasing number of options when considering definitive treatment of VHD. These will include more endovascular approaches and more valve repair. Considering the excellent outcomes and low complication rate of valve surgery in many centers, it seems very unlikely that percutaneous approaches will ever replace open procedures.

# References

Bergler-Klein J, Klaar U, Heger M, *et al.* (2004). Natriuretic peptides predict symptom free survival and postoperative outcome in severe aortic stenosis. *Circulation* **109**:2302–2308.

Boudjemline Y, Agnoletti G, Bonnett D, Sidi D, Bonhoeffer P (2004). Percutaneous pulmonary valve replacement in a large right ventricular outflow tract: an experimental study. *Journal of the American College of Cardiology* **43**:1082–1087.

Bristow MR, Saxon LA, Boehmer J, *et al.* (2004). Cardiac resynchronization therapy with or without an implantable defibrillator in advanced chronic heart failure. *New England Journal of Medicine* **350**:2140–2150.

Caruthers SD, Lin SJ, Brown P, *et al.* (2003). Practical value of cardiac magnetic resonance imaging for clinical quantification of aortic valve stenosis: comparision with echocardiography. *Circulation* **108**:2236–2243.

Chang CP, Neilson JR, Bayle JH, *et al.* (2004). A field of myocardial-endocardial NFAT signaling underlies heart valve morphogenesis. *Cell* **118**:649–663.

Chau KL, Dumesnil JG, Cujec B, *et al.* (2003). A randomized trial of aspirin on the risk of embolic events in patients with infective endocarditis. *Journal of the American College of Cardiology* **42**:775–780.

Cohen G, Christakis GT, Joyner CD, *et al.* (2002). Are stentless valves hemodynamically superior to stented valves? A prospective randomized trial. *Annals of Thoracic Surgery* **73**:767–778.

Cribier A, Eltchaninoff, Tron C, *et al.* (2004). Early experience with percutaneous transcatheter implantation of heart valve prosthesis for the treatment of end-stage inoperable patients with calcific aortic stenosis. *Journal of the American College of Cardiology* **43**:698–703.

Gerber IL, Stewart RAH, Hammett CJK, *et al.* (2003a). Effect of aortic valve replacement on C-reactive protein in nonrheumatic aortic stenosis. *American Journal of Cardiology* **93**:1129–1132.

Gerber IL, Stewart RAH, French JK, *et al.* (2003b). Associations between plasma natriuretic peptide levels, symptoms, and left ventricular function in patients with chronic aortic regurgitation. *American Journal of Cardiology* **92**:755–758.

Grande-Allen KJ, Borowski AG, Trougton RW, *et al.* (2005). Apparently normal mitral valves in patients with heart failure demonstrate biochemical and structural derangements: an extracellular matrix and echocardiographic study. *Journal of the American College of Cardiology* **45**:54–61.

Kaden JJ, Bickelhaupt S, Grobholz R, *et al.* (2004). Expression of bone sialoprotein and bone morphogenetic protein-2 in calcific aortic stenosis. *Journal of Heart Valve Disease* **13**(4):560–566.

Kaye DM, Byrne M, Alferness C, Power J (2003). Feasibility and short-term efficacy of percutaneous mitral annular reduction for the therapy of heart failure-induced mitral regurgitation. *Circulation* **108**:1795–1797.

Lockhart PB, Brennan MT, Louise Kent M, Norton HJ, Weinrib DA (2004). Impact of amoxicillin prophylaxis on the incidence, nature, and duration of bacteremia in children after intubation and dental procedures. *Circulation* **109**:2878–2884.

Mazzone A, Epistolata MC, DeCaterina R, *et al.* (2004). Neoangiogenesis, T-lymphocyte infiltration, and heat shock protein-60 are biological hallmarks of an immunomediated inflammatory process in end-stage calcified aortic valve stenosis. *Journal of the American College of Cardiology* **43**:1670–1676.

Minakata K, Schaff HV, Zehr KJ, *et al.* (2004). Is repair of aortic valve regurgitation a safe alternative to valve replacement? *Journal of Thoracic and Cardiovascular Surgery* **127**:645–653.

Morgan-Hughes AJ, Owens PE, Robottom CJ, Marshall AJ (2003). Three dimensional volume quantification of aortic valve calcification using multislice computed tomography. *Heart* **89**:1191–1194.

Mueller C, Huber P, Laifer G, Mueller B, Perruchoud AP (2004). Procalcitonin and the early diagnosis of infective endocarditis. *Circulation* **109**:1707–1710.

Murday AJ, Hochstizky A, Mansfield J, *et al.* (2003). A prospective controlled trial of St. Jude versus Starr–Edwards aortic and mitral valve prostheses. *Annals of Thoracic Surgery* **76**:66–74.

Nasuti JF, Zhang PJ, Feldman MD, *et al.* (2004). Fibrillin and other matrix proteins in mitral valve prolapse syndrome. *Annals of Thoracic Surgery* 77:532–536.

Nataatmadja M, West M, West J, *et al.* (2003). Abnormal extracelluar matrix protein transport associated with incresed apoptosis of vascular smooth muscle cells in Marfan syndrome and bicuspid aortic valve thoracic aortic aneurysms. *Circulation* 108(Supplement II):329–334.

Navaro GM, Sachar R, Pearce GL, Sprecher DL, Griffin BP (2003). Association between apolipoprotein E alleles and calcific valvular disease. *Circulation* 108:1804–1808.

Ohashi KL, Culkar J, Riebman JB, Estes M, Constantz BR, Yoganathan AP (2004). Hemodynamic characterization of calcified stenotic human aortic valves before and after treatment with a novel aortic valve repair system. *Journal of Heart Valve Disease* 13(4):582–592.

Pu M, Thomas JD, Gillinor MA, Griffin BP, Brunken RC (2003). Importance of ischemic and viable myocardium for patients with chronic ischemic mitral regurgitation and left ventricular dysfunction. *American Journal of Cardiology* 92:862–864.

Rahimtoola SH (2005). The year in valvular heart disease. *Journal of the American College of Cardiology* 45(1):111–122.

Rajamannan NM, Subramaniam M, Rickard D, *et al.* (2003). Human aortic valve calcification is associated with an osteoblast phenotype. *Circulation* 107(17):2181–2184.

St. Goar FG, Fann JL, Komtebbedde J, *et al.* (2003). Endovascular edge-to-edge mitral valve repair: short term results in a porcine model. *Circulation* 108:1990–1993.

Satta J, Oliva J, Salo T, *et al.* (2003). Evidence of altered balance between matrix metalloproteinase-9 and its inhibitors in calcific aortic stenosis. *Annals of Thoracic Surgery* 76:681–688.

Shworak NW (2004). Angiogenic modulators in valve development and disease: does valvular disease recapitulate developmental signaling pathways? *Current Opinions in Cardiology* 19(2):140–146.

Teshima H, Hayashida N, Fukunaga S, *et al.* (2004). Usefulness of computed tomography scanner for detecting pannus formation. *Annals of Thoracic Surgery* 7:523–526.

Walsh CR, Larson MG, Kupka MJ, *et al.* (2004). Association of aortic valve calcium detected by electron beam computed tomography with echocardiographic aortic valve disease and with calcium deposits in the coronary arteries and thoracic aorta. *Journal of the American College of Cardiology* 93:421–425.

Young JB, Abraham WT, Smith AL, *et al.* (2003). Combined cardiac resynchronization and implantable cardioversion defibrillation in advanced chronic heart failure: the MIRACLE ICD Trial. *Journal of the American Medical Association* 289:2685–2694.

Zamorano J, Cordeiro P, Sugeng L, *et al.* (2004). Real-time three dimensional echocardiography for rheumatic mitral stenosis evaluation: an accurate and novel approach. *Journal of the American College of Cardiology* 43:2091–2096.

# Appendix A

# Seminal Randomized Clinical Trials in Valvular Heart Disease

## Prevention

Olsen MH, Wachtell K, Bella JN, *et al.* (2004). Effect of losartan versus atenolol on aortic valve sclerosis (a LIFE substudy). *American Journal of Cardiology* **94**(8):1076–1080.

*This was a substudy of the LIFE trial, a study comparing the effects of atenolol and losartan in eldery, hypertensive patients. The data failed to show any difference in the rate of progression in aortic sclerosis in the two arms of the trial.*

Raggi P, Bommer J, Chertow GM (2004). Valvular calcification in hemodialysis patients randomized to calcium-based phosphorus binders or sevelamer. *Journal of Heart Valve Disease* **13**(1):134–141.

*In this randomized trial from Tulane University, 200 patients on maintenance hemodialysis were randomized to sevelamer or calcium-based phosphorus binders. Electron beam computed tomography of the coronary arteries and heart valves was performed at baseline and at 1 year. There was a trend towards reduced progression of mitral and combined mitral and aortic calcification in the sevelamer treated group. When vascular and valvular calcification scores were combined, the differences in progression were statistically significant. More patients in the sevelamer arm achieved arrest or regression in total vascular and valvular calcification.*

## Prosthetic valves

Murday AJ, Hochstitzky A, Mansfield J, *et al.* (2003). A prospective controlled trial of St. Jude versus Starr–Edwards aortic and mitral valve prostheses. *Annals of Thoracic Surgery* **76**(1):66–73.

*In this prospective randomized trial from St. George's Hospital in London, 389 patients undergoing mechanical valve replacement in the mitral or aortic position were randomized to a St. Jude or Starr–Edwards prosthesis. The authors found no difference in the rates of complication or symptomatic improvement in either valve position.*

Oxenham H, Bloomfield P, Wheatley DJ, *et al.* (2003). Twenty year comparison of Bjork–Shiley mechanical heart valve with porcine bioprothesis. *Heart* **89**(7):715–721.

*This publication by the Royal Infirmary of Edinburgh, reports the follow-up of patients randomized to a Bjork–Shiley or a porcine prosthesis between 1975 and 1979. Using the combined endpoint of death and reoperation, there appears to be improved outcomes among patients receiving the Bjork–Shiley prosthesis. The two groups diverged by 8–10 years for mitral replacement and by 12–14 years for aortic valve replacement. Major bleeding was more common in patients receiving the mechanical valve with its attendant requirement for anticoagulation.*

Autschbach R, Walther T, Falk V, *et al.* (2000). Prospectively randomized comparison of different mechanical aortic valves. *Circulation* **102**(19 Supplement 3):III 1–4.

*This study from Leipzeig, Germany compared outcomes of death, stroke, reoperation, valve incompetence, paravalvular leak, flow velocities, and ventricular hypertrophy in 300 consecutive patients randomized to ATS, Carbomedics, and St. Jude Medical Hemodynamic Plus mechanical valves in the aortic position. At 1 year, there were no differences in any of these rates among the 100 patients assigned to each arm of the study.*

Aklog L, Carr-White GS, Birks EJ, Yacoub MH (2000). Pulmonary autograft versus aortic homograft for aortic valve replacement: interim results from a prospective randomized trial. *Journal of Heart Valve Disease* **9**(2):176–188.

*This publication from the Royal Brompton-Harefield NHS Trust, UK, reports the most recent interim analysis of a prospective randomized trial of 182 patients randomized to pulmonary autograft versus homograft aortic valve replacement. Patients undergoing autograft had longer cross-clamp and bypass times. At a median follow-up of 33.9 months, there was no difference in actuarial and reoperation-free survival. Echocardiography was interpreted as showing early signs of subclinical dysfunction in many of the homografts. The results of subsequent follow-up are eagerly awaited.*

## Atrial fibrillation

Jessurun ER, van Hemel NM, Defau JJ, *et al.* (2003). A randomized study of combining maze surgery for atrial fibrillation with mitral valve surgery. *Journal of Cardiovascular Surgery* **44**(1):9–18.

*In this trial from St. Anonius Hospital in the Netherlands, 35 patients with atrial fibrillation (AF) undergoing mitral valve surgery were randomized in a 2.5:1 ratio to surgery with, versus without a Maze III procedure. The primary endpoint was freedom from AF and follow-up was a minimum of 1 year. At 12 months follow-up, freedom from AF was 92% vs. 20% in the Maze and no Maze groups respectively. Stroke was observed in one patient in the no Maze group. There was no difference in quality of life measures in the two groups.*

## Mitral valvuloplasty

Bhat A, Harikrishan S, Tharakan JM, *et al.* (2002). Comparison of percutaneous transmitral commissurotomy with Inoue balloon technique and metallic commissurotomy: immediate and short-term follow-up results of a randomized study. *American Heart Journal* **144**(6):1074–1080.

*This study from Kerala, India, compared the outcomes of 100 patients with mitral stenosis randomized to percutaneous transmitral commissurotomy by Inoue balloon or metallic commissurotomy. Procedural success, complication rate, and hemodynamic parameters were all equal at 4 months of follow-up.*

## Infective endocarditis

Schaff HV, Carrel TP, Jamieson WRE, *et al.* (2002). Paravalvular leak and other events in Silzone-coated mechanical heart valves: a report from AVERT. *Annals of Thoracic Surgery* **73**(3):785–792.

*The Artificial Valve Endocarditis Reduction Trial (AVERT) was an international multicenter randomized clinical trial initiated in 1999 which sought to enroll 4400 patients in 17 centers in North America and Europe, to compare the efficacy of a Silizone coating versus no coating on the sewing cuff of a St. Jude Medical Masters Series mechanical valve in the prevention of infective endocarditis. However, the trial was terminated in February 2000 after the enrolment of 807 patients, because of an apparent increased risk of perivalvular leak in the Silizone-coated arm of the trial. This trial shares the name (AVERT) of a later trial which evaluated the effect of intensive lipid lowering therapy on coronary atherosclerosis.*

Herijgers P, Herrogods MC, Vandeplas A, Meyns B, Flameng W (2001). Silzone coating and peravalvular leak: an independent, randomized study. *Journal of Heart Valve Disease* **10**(6):712–715.

*As in the AVERT trial, this study compared outcomes in a separate population of 95 patients randomized to Silzone-coated versus uncoated St. Jude Medical Masters prostheses. In echocardiographic follow-up averaging 478 +/- 78 days, there were no major paravalvular leaks seen. Five of 51 coated valves had minimal or slight paravalvular leak compared to 3 of 53 uncoated valves. Serum LDH (an indicator of hemolysis) was 654 in the coated group and 598 in the uncoated group. Neither of these differences were statistically significant.*

# Appendix B

# International Websites Relevant to Valvular Heart Disease

**Academic and Specialty Societies**
American Heart Association
http://www.americanheart.org
American College of Cardiology
http://www.acc.org
American Society of Echocardiography
http://asecho.org
American Association for Thoracic Surgery
http://www.aats.org
Asian Society for Cardiovascular Surgery
http://www.ascvs.org
British Cardiac Society
http://www.bcs.com
Brazilian Society of Cardiology
http://www.cardiol.br
Canadian Cardiovascular Society
http://www.ccs.ca
Cardiac Society of Australia and New Zealand
http://www.csanz.edu.au
European Association for Cardiothoracic Surgery
http://www.eacts.org
European Association of Echocardiography
http://www.escardio.org/bodies/associations/EAE
European Society of Cardiology
http://www.escardio.org
Heart Valve Society of America
http://www.heartvalvesocietyofamerica.org
Society for Heart Valve Disease.
http://www.shvd.org
Society of Thoracic Surgeons
http://www.sts.org

**Prosthetic heart valve manufacturers**
Boston Scientific
http://www.bostonscientific.com
CarboMedics  (subsidiary of Sorin)
http://www.carbomedics.com
Edwards Lifesciences
http://www.edwards.com
Guidant
http://www.guidant.com

Medtronics
http://www.medtronic.com
St. Jude Medical
http://www.sjm.com

**Intraaortic balloon pumps and insertion kits**
Arrow International
http://www.arrowintl.com
Datascope
http://www.datascope.com

**Vavlotomy balloon catheters**
Toray
http://www.torayusa.com

**Echocardiography and magnetic resonance manufacturers**
GE Healthcare
http://www.gehealthcare.com
Philips Medical Systems
http://www.medical.philips.com
Siemens Medical
http://www.medical.siemens.com

**Electronic stethoscopes**
Andromed
http://www.andromed.com
Cardionics
http://www.cardionics.com
Philips Medical Systems
http://www.medical.philips.com
Stethographics
http://www.stethographics.com
3M Healthcare (Littmann)
http://www.3m.com/us/healthcare
Welch Allyn
http://www.welchallyn.com/medical

**Patient education**
American Heart Association-Patient Information
http://www.americanheart.org
European Society of Cardiology-Patient Information
http://www.escardio.org/knowledge/links/
patients.htm

# Index